SHARON

D060725

SHARON

PERIODONTAL DISEASE:

CLINICAL, RADIOGRAPHIC
AND
HISTOPATHOLOGIC FEATURES

IRVING GLICKMAN, B.S., D.M.D., F.A.C.D., F.I.C.D.

*Late Professor and Chairman of the Department of Periodontology;
Research Professor of Oral Pathology, Tufts University School of
Dental Medicine, Boston, Massachusetts*

JEROME B. SMULOW, A.B., D.D.S., M.S., F.A.C.D.

*Professor of Periodontology, Tufts University School of Dental
Medicine, Boston, Massachusetts*

W. B. SAUNDERS COMPANY • PHILADELPHIA • LONDON • TORONTO   1974

W. B. Saunders Company: West Washington Square
Philadelphia, PA 19105

12 Dyott Street
London, WC1A 1DB

833 Oxford Street
Toronto, Ontario M8Z   5T9, Canada

Library of Congress Cataloging in Publication Data

Glickman, Irving and Smulow, Jerome B.

Periodontal disease: clinical, radiographic, and histopathologic
features.

1. Periodontal disease.   I. Smulow, Jerome B., joint author.
   II. Title.   [DNLM: 1. Periodontal diseases.   WU240
   G559p 1974]

RK361.G582   617.6'32   71-145558
ISBN 0-7216-4138-5

Periodontal Disease   ISBN   0-7216-4138-5

© 1974 by W. B. Saunders Company. Copyright under the International Copyright Union.
All rights reserved. This book is protected by copyright. No part of it may be reproduced,
stored in a retrieval system, or transmitted in any form or by any means, electronic, mechanical,
photocopying, recording, or otherwise, without written permission from the publisher. Made
in the United States of America. Press of W. B. Saunders Company. Library of Congress
catalog card number 71-145558.

Last digit is the print number: 9   8   7   6   5   4   3   2   1

Dedication and Memoriam

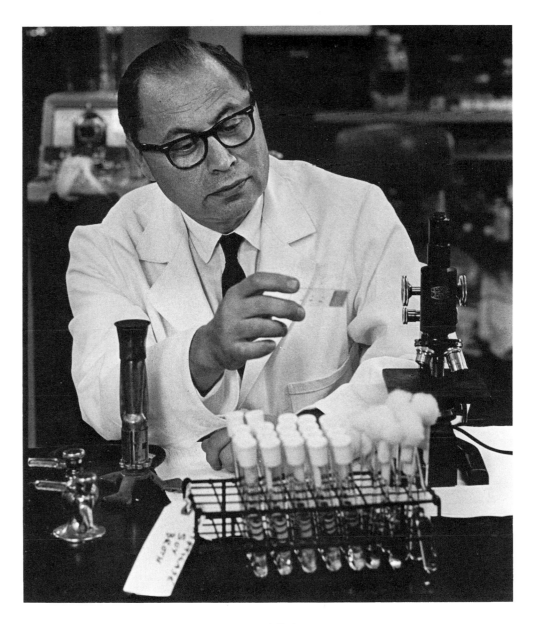

Irving Glickman
1914–1972

my teacher and dear friend, whose constant stimulation, enormous energy and unbounded enthusiasm provided the impetus for the initiation, development and completion of this work. His scholarly achievements and the memory of his perceptive and questioning mind will continue to guide us.

Preface

This concise pictorial text is intended to provide a guide for those interested in understanding and diagnosing gingival and periodontal disease. Clinical, radiographic, and histologic photographs are compared in a large, easily interpreted format. Subject units are succinct, generally one or two pages in length. Together they comprise a comprehensive summary of the field. A section on experimental pathology is included to give the reader a realization of the importance of the laboratory in generating scientifically based knowledge which is necessary for the development of practical clinical concepts.

We are indebted to our colleagues at Tufts University School of Dental Medicine, Dr. Frank Susi, Department of Oral Biology, for the preparation of the electron photomicrographs and Dr. Samuel Turesky, Department of Periodontology, for his suggestions in the areas of plaque and calculus formation. Credit must go to Mr. Leo Goodman and Mr. Martin Snyder, photographers at the Mallory Institute of Pathology, Boston City Hospital, for their excellent photographic work. Recognition is due Mr. Robert Ullrich, Medical Illustrator, Tufts University Schools of Medicine and Dental Medicine, for his fine artwork; and the staff at W. B. Saunders Company for their cooperation and attention to detail. Special appreciation goes to Rachel Hill for preparation of the histopathologic material and Janice El Qudsi for her secretarial assistance.

It falls upon me to express to Violeta Glickman, just as I express to my wife, Miriam, my thanks and gratitude for their encouragement throughout the preparation of this book. Finally, I wish to acknowledge the contribution of my co-author, the late Dr. Irving Glickman, who shared with me the arduous labor of this work.

JEROME B. SMULOW
BOSTON, MASS.

Contents

Experimental Pathology

GINGIVAL PIGMENTATION

Melanin is an endogenous pigment commonly observed in the skin and oral tissues of dark skinned individuals. It is also found in lesser amounts in persons with fair complexions. Other tissues, such as the retina of the eye, also contain melanin. In the mouth, the gingiva and hard palate are the most frequently pigmented tissues. Melanin is produced in cells called melanocytes which are found primarily in the basal cell layer of the epithelium. The amino acid, tyrosine is the precursor of melanin. In the presence of the enzyme tryosinase, tyrosine is converted to DOPA (dioxyphenylalanine), which then goes through a series of chemical reactions to become melanin, a granular pigment that varies in color from yellow-brown to black. The pigment granules are deposited in macrophages within the connective tissue called melanophages (melanophores). These cells carry the pigment but do not produce it. Melanin granules are also found in the cytoplasm of epithelial cells, primarily those of the basal layer.

When pigmented gingival tissue is removed surgically as in gingivectomy, the newly formed gingiva is not pigmented. The pigment often does not return but when it does, it comes back slowly and in lesser amounts.

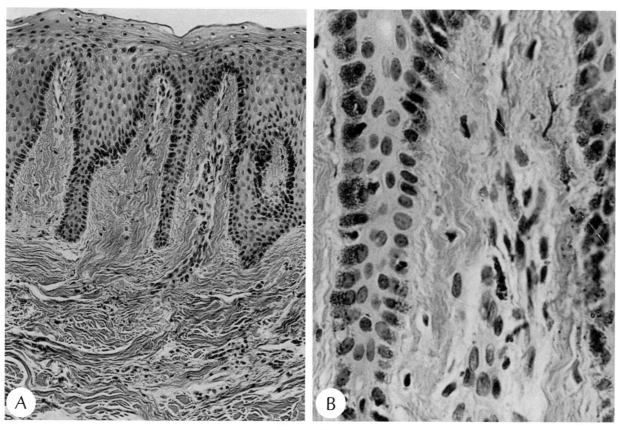

Figure 2

A. Biopsy taken from individual shown in Fig. 1B. Indentations on the surface represent stippling. The epithelium is parakeratotic and numerous pigmented cells containing melanin granules are seen in the basal layer. Cells containing melanin granules (melanophages) are present in the connective tissue. The collagen fibers are numerous and well formed.

B. When the tissue seen in Fig. 2A is examined at higher power the melanin granules in the pigmented cells of both epithelium and connective tissue are more readily apparent. A few chronic inflammatory cells are present in the connective tissue.

Figure 3. See illustration on opposite page.

Serial sections of marginal and attached gingiva stained by different techniques to demonstrate structural components. Fig. 3A. Hematoxylin and Eosin stain for normal histologic detail. Fig. 3B. Mallory Connective Tissue stain to demonstrate collagen fibers. Fig. 3C. Periodic acid-Schiff reaction for glycogen. Fig. 3D. Periodic acid-Schiff reaction treated with diastase to remove glycogen. Fig. 3E. High power of epithelial cells stained with Toluidine Blue to demonstrate staining of intercellular bridges and absence of staining between bridges. Fig. 3F. Astrablau counterstained with Neutral Red to demonstrate blue staining granules in mast cells.

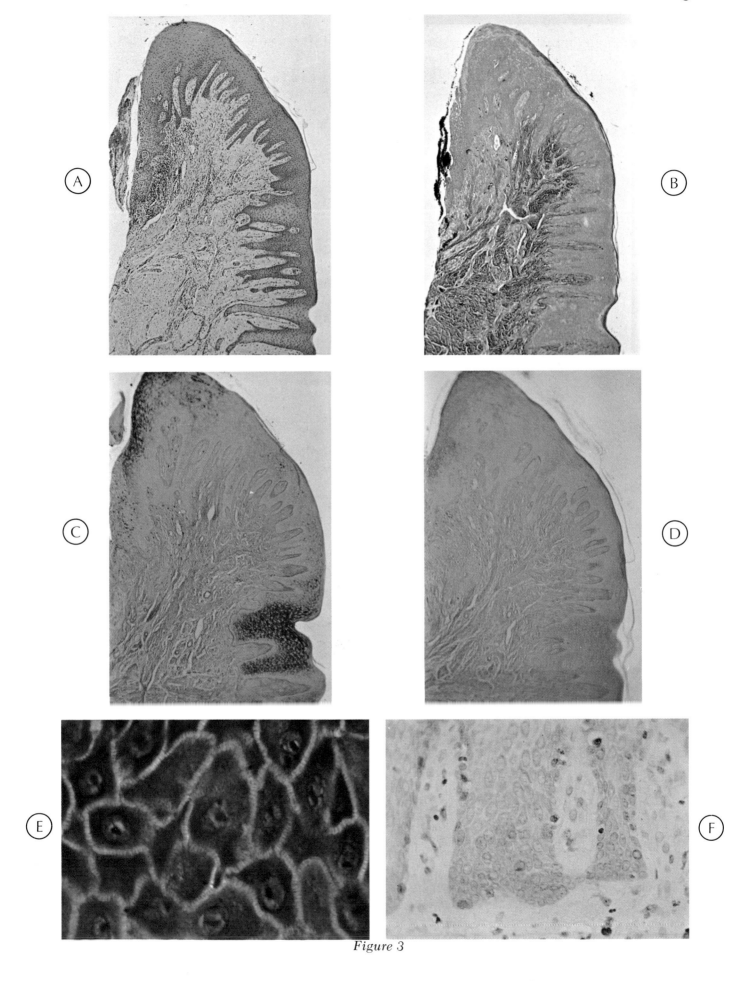

Figure 3

Gingival Fibers

The bulk of the connective tissue of the gingiva is composed of collagen fibers. These fibers provide strength and rigidity to the tissue and help it withstand the forces of mastication. The fibers are fairly thick (about the same diameter as red blood cells) and are composed of smaller units called fibrils and microfibrils. Collagen fibers have great tensile strength. They do not stretch like elastic fibers but because they are often wavy, can be extended. Collagen is the most common protein found in the body. It is composed of eighteen amino acids, two of which, hydroxyproline and hydroxylysine are unique to collagen. Because of this, the amount of hydroxyproline found in a tissue is often used as a measure of its collagen content.

The collagen fibers of the gingiva can be subdivided into large groups based on their location. The largest group is the gingivodental fibers. These fibers are embedded in the cementum of the tooth and extend into the tissue in three directions: occlusally into the gingival margin; apically over the crest of the alveolar bone; and horizontally into the gingiva. The circular fibers form the second major subdivision. These surround the tooth in a ring or collar-like fashion. They are less numerous than the gingivodental fibers and are more difficult to demonstrate histologically. They help to hold the gingiva tightly against the tooth. The third type or subdivision is the transseptal fibers which are seen in mesio-distal sections. They extend from tooth to tooth over the crest of the alveolar bone. Some suggest that the transseptal fibers should be considered part of the periodontal ligament rather than grouped with the gingival fibers.

Other fibers are found in the gingival connective tissue but in much lesser amounts. Reticular fibers are a protein, chemically similar to collagen, and when examined with the electron microscope, they reveal the same axial periodicity. It has been suggested that they represent an immature precursor to collagen. They are differentiated from collagen by their finer structure and different staining characteristics, for example, they stain more deeply with silver (argyrophilic) and periodic acid-Schiff (magenta) than does collagen. Reticular fibers form a network located just beneath the epithelium where they contribute to the connective tissue portion of the basement lamina. Elastic fibers are found in the gingiva but these are rare and seen mainly in relation to blood vessels. A fourth type, called oxytalan fibers, has also been described. These, too, are uncommon and require special histochemical staining techniques for their demonstration. Oxytalan fibers may be related in some way to elastic fibers, possibly an immature form.

All of the fibers and cells found in the gingival tissue are embedded in a viscous ground substance consisting principally of polysaccharide and protein compounds called mucopolysaccharides. These large molecular weight substances which are essentially carbohydrates with an attached protein fraction are divided into those which are non-sulfated such as hyaluronic acid and its isomer chondroitin and those which are sulfated such as chondroitin sulfate A, B, and C. They are all colloids and as such, help to regulate the distribution of water, electrolytes and metabolites in the tissues. Glycoproteins, basically proteins with an added carbohydrate group, are also found in the gingival ground substance.

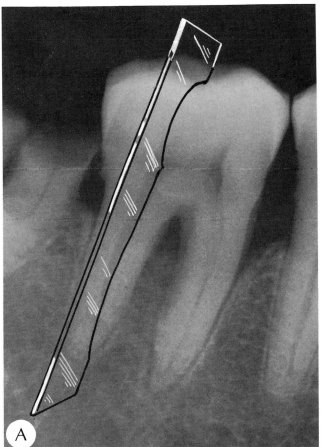

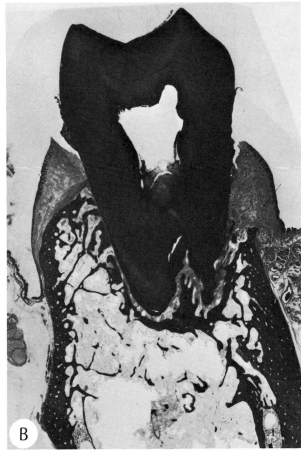

A. Radiograph of mandibular second molar area. There is bifurcation involvement with reduction in bone height and slight funnel-shaped widening of the periodontal ligament on the mesial and distal. The glass cut indicates the plane of section shown in (B).

B. Bucco-lingual section of mandibular second molar shown in (A). There is considerable bone loss on the buccal (right) which is not readily apparent in the radiograph. The long axis of the tooth is directed lingually.

C. Higher power of lingual gingiva and crest of bone seen in (B). The gingival fibers are well formed. They pass from the cementum apically over the crest of bone and coronally toward the gingival crest. As a result of inflammation the epithelium lining the pocket is thinned and ulcerated. A mass of calculus can be seen attached to the tooth in this area.

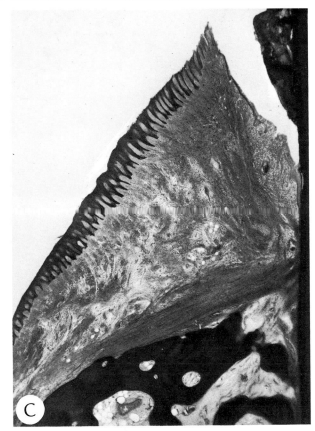

Figure 6

GINGIVAL SULCUS

The gingival sulcus is a small triangular space or potential space whose apex points rootward. It is bounded on one side by the tooth and on the other by the sulcular epithelium. The most commonly held concept of sulcus formation is that after enamel formation (amelogenesis) is complete, the ameloblasts, which produce the enamel, then form the primary enamel cuticle, a calcified structure which covers the crown of the tooth. All of the epithelial cells, inner enamel epithelium (ameloblasts), stellate reticulum, stratum intermedium, and outer enamel epithelium, which took part in the formation of the enamel organ are compressed to a few layers of cuboidal cells called the reduced enamel epithelium. The reduction of these layers takes place at different times, the stellate reticulum being reduced and disappearing earliest. The reduced ameloblasts remain organically attached to the enamel. As the tooth erupts and approaches the surface, the reduced enamel epithelium covering the crown of the tooth fuses with the epithelium lining the oral cavity. When the tooth penetrates into the oral cavity, the area where the reduced enamel epithelium fuses with the oral epithelium becomes the marginal gingiva. The space between the tooth and the marginal gingiva is called the sulcus, and the reduced enamel epithelium which is attached to the crown of the tooth becomes the epithelial attachment. When the tooth first enters the mouth, the root is still not fully formed and continues to develop as the tooth erupts. At the time the tooth meets its occlusal antagonist about one-third of the anatomical crown is still below the gingiva. Some investigators suggest that the gingival sulcus forms from a split within the epithelium rather than by a progressive separation of the coronal portion of the entire epithelial attachment from the tooth surface. More recently, other workers have maintained that the cells of the epithelial attachment are not really attached to the tooth but are just firmly compressed against it forming a collar. Recent electron microscopic studies have shown that in humans the reduced ameloblasts and gingival epithelial cells which comprise the epithelial attachment form a very fine basement lamina structure on the enamel and cementum. Hemidesmosomes are produced by these cells and attach the epithelium to this lamina. This seems to support the concept that the cells of the epithelial attachment are organically bound to the tooth.

Ideally, the sulcus depth would be zero and not permit entry of even a fine probe. In reality, the sulcus usually measures about one to two millimeters in depth. In humans, the eipthelium lining the sulcus is non-keratinized and does not contain rete pegs. The reverse is true of the epithelium lining the facial surface of the marginal gingiva. In monkeys, autoradiographic studies using tritiated thymidine have shown that in health the epithelial cells comprising the epithelial attachment are less active as measured by uptake of labelling than the epithelial cells lining the sulcus or the facial surface of the gingiva. However, when there is inflammation present, the cells of the epithelial attachment become more active than those of the other two areas. This increase in activity in the epithelial attachment might accelerate the apical migration of the epithelium on the tooth surface.

The gingival sulcus is critical to the health of the gingiva because local irritants that initiate gingival inflammation accumulate there. The sulcus is bathed by a fluid (gingival fluid), which seeps into it from the gingiva. This fluid, whose composition is similar to that of serum, may be protective in that it washes particulate matter from the sulcus. It contains immunoglobulins and granulocytes and is antimicrobial. Inflammation increases the flow of gingival fluid.

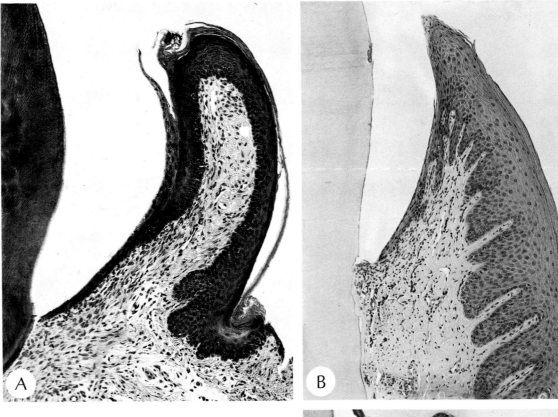

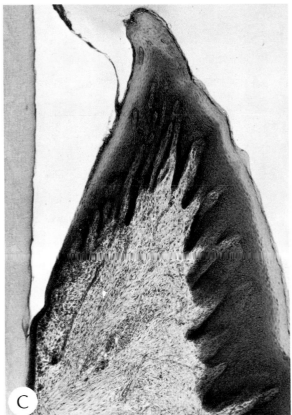

A. Rat sulcus with base of epithelial attachment at cemento-enamel junction. The sulcus is lined with enamel epithelium which is being undermined by the thicker oral epithelium. Note that in the rat the sulcular surface is keratinized. The connective tissue contains some leukocytes.

B. Dog sulcus with base of epithelial attachment located at cemento-enamel junction. There is a slight infiltration of inflammatory cells beneath the sulcular epithelium. The oral epithelium is proliferating and replaces the enamel epithelium. The sulcular wall is non-keratinized.

C. Monkey sulcus with inflammatory infiltrate in the connective tissue. The epithelial attachment has proliferated along the cementum and the epithelium lining the sulcus is hyperplastic. The strand-like structure projecting from the sulcular epithelium is a remnant of the enamel cuticle.

Figure 7

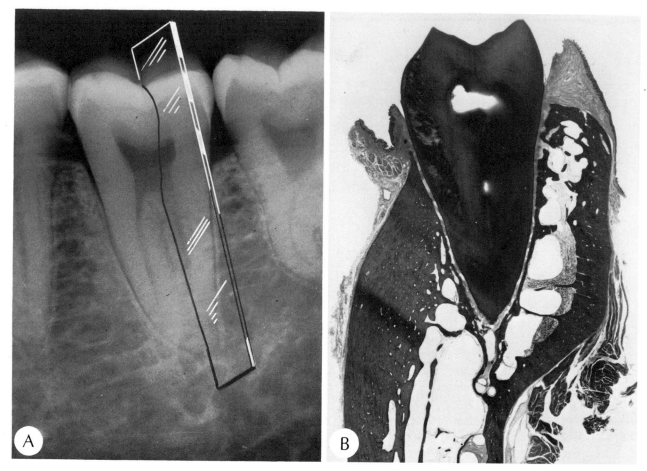

Figure 8

A. Radiograph of mandibular molar area. There is funnel-shaped widening of the peri-odontal ligament space mesial to the second molar. The glass cut indicates the plane of section shown in Fig. 8B.

B. Bucco-lingual section of mandible through second molar shown in Fig. 8A. The cortical plates both buccally (left) and lingually (right) are very dense.

Illustration continued on opposite page.

CUTICLES

The primary or enamel cuticle is a thin acellular structure less than one micron thick covering the crown of the newly erupted tooth. It is calcified and believed to be formed from or by the ameloblasts after enamel matrix production ceases. It develops in direct continuity with the enamel matrix and is therefore not merely adjacent to the enamel but in organic union with it. The primary cuticle is found to be somewhat more resistant to acids and alkalies than the enamel. It is quickly worn off exposed tooth surfaces by the abrasive action of foods during chewing. However, it can be found in protected areas such as the gingival sulcus, developmental grooves, and the interproximal areas of the tooth.

There is another cuticle which covers not only the crown of the tooth but also the exposed portion of the root. This cuticle is known as the secondary cuticle (dental

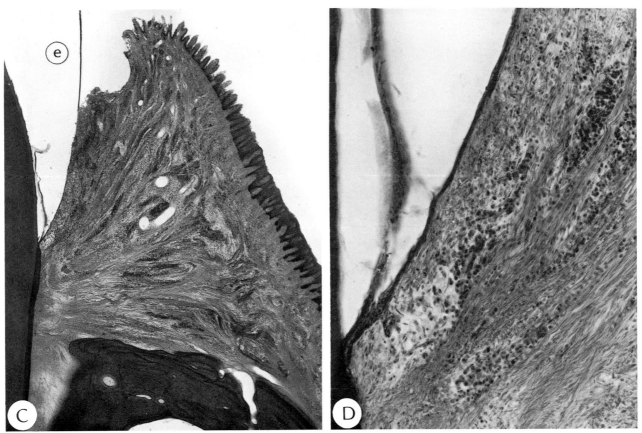

Figure 8

Legend continued.

C. Higher power of lingual gingiva and crest of bone shown in Fig. 8B. The gingival tissue is infiltrated with leukocytes; however, as yet there is no bone loss. The periodontal ligament is slightly widened in the coronal portion. The epithelial attachment and the enamel cuticle are both located at the cemento-enamel junction. The enamel (e) has been dissolved in preparation of the section.

D. High power of sulcular area shown in Fig. 8C. The epithelial attachment is quite thin with the exception of an area in close proximity to the cemento-enamel junction where there is a bud of proliferating epithelium. The connective tissue is infiltrated with leukocytes and is edematous in the area of the proliferating epithelium. The enamel cuticle is attached at the cemento-enamel junction and can be seen in the space formerly occupied by the tooth enamel.

cuticle or cuticular dentis). It is found on most but not all teeth. On the crown of the tooth, the primary and secondary cuticles fuse forming a single structure (Nasmyth's membrane). The secondary cuticle is a non-calcified, non-keratinized protein-carbohydrate substance. It is believed to be elaborated by the cells of the epithelial attachment and deposited on the tooth surface exposed by these cells as they migrate apically. It has also been suggested that substances from the saliva, gingival fluid and blood cells contribute to its composition. The secondary cuticle is found on the cementum of teeth only in areas which are or have been covered by cells from the epithelial attachment. It is not found where the periodontal ligament fibers are embedded in the cementum. As with the primary cuticle, it is rapidly worn off exposed tooth surfaces but may be found in protected areas.

Electron Microscopy — Normal and Inflamed Gingiva

The electron microscope provides a means for examination of tissue at much higher magnification than that which is obtainable from a regular light microscope. The overall picture of the tissue is unobtainable in one view, but this is compensated for by the increased detail seen in the area being studied.

Sections of clinically normal gingival tissue were examined under the electron microscope and compared with chronically inflamed gingiva. The following epithelial and connective tissue structures were demonstrated in both the clinically normal and diseased tissue and are illustrated on the following pages: spinous and basal cell layers of the epithelium, basement lamina and lamina propria of the connective tissue.

In health, typical stratum spinosum cells exhibit a somewhat spherical outline and a round, centrally-placed nucleus (Fig. 9A). Similar cytoplasmic organelles are present as in the stratum basale. Tonofilaments of about 80-90Å in width are present in increased numbers, forming large bundles which appear to surround the nuclei and then approach, and possibly fuse with desmosomal attachment plaques peripherally. Desmosomes are more numerous and somewhat larger than in the stratum basale, but are of similar architecture (Fig. 9B). Each attachment plaque is approximately 150Å in thickness and of variable length, ranging between 400-500 mμ. The intervening intercellular space measures 300-350Å and contains seven layers parallel to one another. The center of the space is occupied by a dense layer of approximately 40-50Å, termed the "intercellular contact layer" (ICL). On either side of the ICL, there is a "distal light layer" of 50-65Å thickness and this in turn is adjacent to the "dense intermediate layer" which measures 35-40Å in width. The intermediate layer, also called the "lateral dense line," is separated from the attachment plaque by a 40-50Å thick, "proximal light layer." The "dense intermediate layer" appears to be continuous with the outer leaflet of the trilaminar cell membrane. In the upper layers of the stratum spinosum, the cells become flattened, with their longer diameter parallel to the basal lamina. In this region the tonofilaments also tend to become oriented in a similar direction.

Figure 9. See illustration on opposite page.

A. Stratum spinosum of clinically normal human gingiva. Typical stratum spinosum cells are spherical with a large central nucleus (n). Tonofilaments (t) are present in high numbers forming larger bundles than in the basal cells. These bundles approach and fuse with desmosomes (d) peripherally. (8,000 ×).

B. Desmosomes of stratum spinosum cut in various planes. Each desmosome consists of two dense attachment plaques (d), to which tonofilaments (t) appear to attach. The intervening space contains three dense layers and four less dense layers. The middle dense layer is the intercellular contact layer. On either side of this layer are the distal light layers which in turn are adjacent to the lateral dense lines. The lateral dense line is separated from the attachment plaque by the proximal light layer. (105,000 ×).

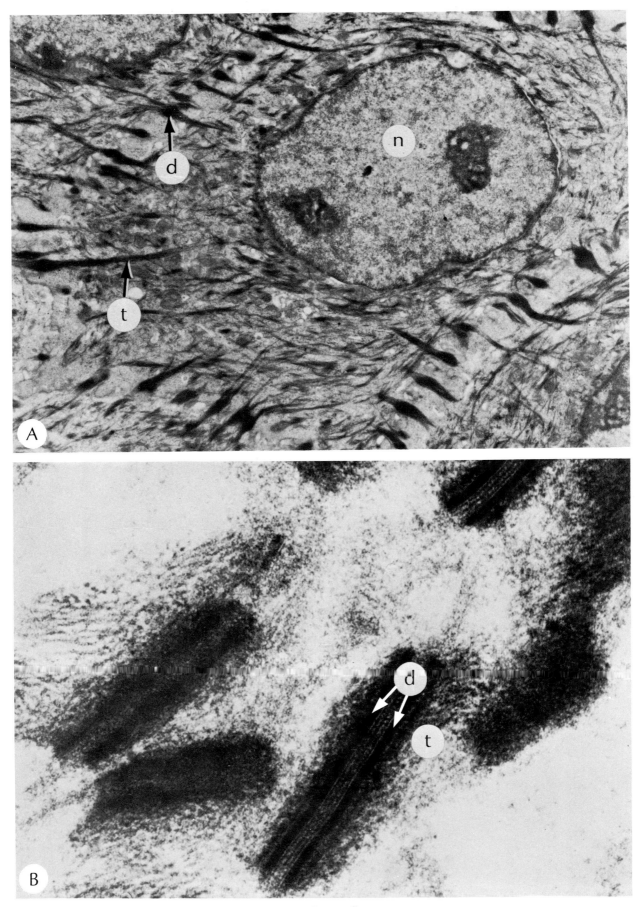

Figure 9

ELECTRON MICROSCOPY — NORMAL AND INFLAMED GINGIVA

The stratum basale consists of a single layer of low columnar cells containing a large centrally- or basally-placed, oval nucleus and cytoplasm containing various organelles, vesicles and filaments. Mitochondria are found mainly in the infranuclear cytoplasm, with a few present at the lateral borders of the nucleus. Endoplasmic reticulum is not well developed and appears as small patches of membrane, studded with ribosomes. Free ribosomes are numerous throughout the cytoplasm. A few smooth-walled, elongated saccules near the superior pole of the nucleus constitute the poorly developed Golgi complex. Smooth-walled, round vesicles are noted at the cell membrane adjacent to the basal lamina. Centrioles may appear in the plane of section adjacent to the superior pole of the nucleus. The most characteristic feature of the cytoplasm of the basal cell is tonofilaments, 60-70Å in diameter and of various lengths, coursing in random fashion or in bundles in a direction perpendicular to the surface of the epithelium.

The cell membrane exhibits a trilaminar unit membrane structure and measures about 75Å in thickness. At the basal lamina side, the cell membrane is quite tortuous enveloping the irregular projections of the cell into the connective tissue. Between adjacent basal cells, the cell membranes are rather straight, becoming quite irregular and wavy again where the basal cells come into contact with spinous cells. Along the lateral and superior surfaces of basal cells, well developed desmosomes appear at areas where adjacent cell membranes are in closest proximity. In general, the intercellular space between basal cells is not very prominent.

Each desmosome consists of two dense attachment plaques located opposite each other at the cytoplasmic side of the adjacent cell membranes. In the 250-350Å space between attachment plaques, seven alternating dense and opaque lines are situated parallel to the cell membrane. These are described in detail under the stratum spinosum. Bundles of tonofilaments appear to run from the attachment plaque into the central cytoplasm of the cell. At the basal lamina side, the cell membrane exhibits half-desmosomes or hemidesmosomes (Fig. 11A). These consist of one attachment plaque without a similar opposing structure. Tonofilaments appear to attach to the cytoplasmic surface of the plaque. Below each hemidesmosome, a thin dense lamella, 60Å thick and corresponding to the central dense lamella of desmosomes, is located in the lamina lucida.

In chronic marginal gingivitis the most obvious alteration in the spinous and basal layers is an increase in the size of the intercellular space (Fig. 10A). Although quantitative studies have not been done, the impression is that there is a decrease in the number of desmosomes per cell. The desmosomes present, however, do not appear markedly altered in morphology (Fig. 10B). Some of the organelles of the epithelial cells may show signs of degeneration such as mitochondrial swelling. Glycogen granules are occasionally observed in the cytoplasm of these cells.

Figure 10. See illustration on opposite page.

A. Cells of the stratum spinosum of chronically inflamed gingiva. Large intercellular spaces (s) are quite evident. Cytoplasmic constituents (tonofilaments, etc.) appear less well organized than in the normal. Compare with Fig. 9A (7,000 ×).

B. Typical desmosomes of the stratum spinosum of chronically inflamed gingiva. The intercellular spaces (s) are quite large in this area. Cellular projections containing tonofilaments (t) can be seen ending in desmosomal (d) structures which do not appear greatly altered. (22,000 ×).

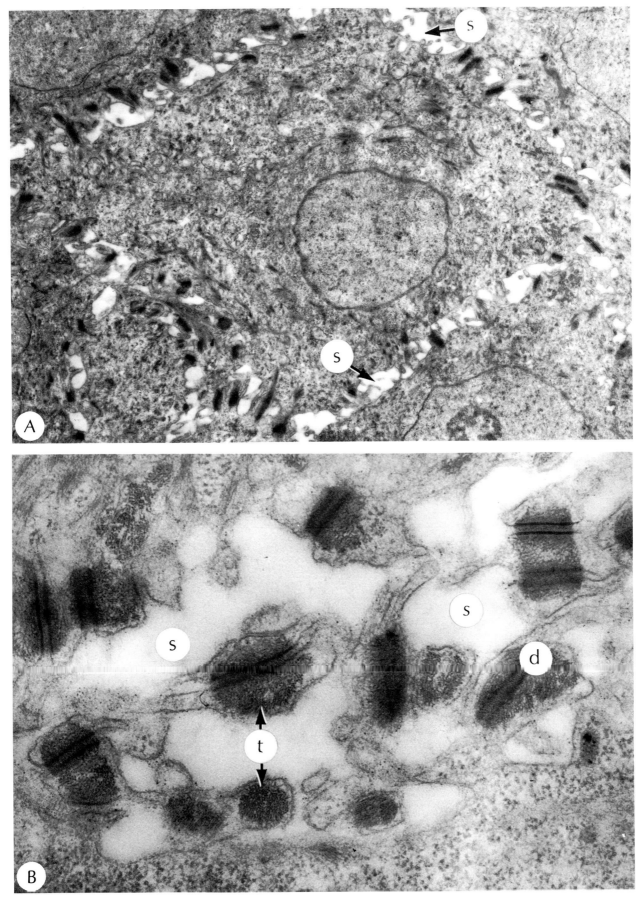

Figure 10

Electron Microscopy—Normal and Inflamed Gingiva

The basal lamina (basement membrane) of clinically normal gingiva consists of an electron-dense layer, the lamina densa, 350-500Å thick, which closely follows basal cell contours and is separated from basal cells by an electron-opaque layer, the lamina lucida, 350-500Å thick (Fig. 11A). At higher magnifications the lamina densa can be seen to consist of fine, dense filaments embedded in a less dense amorphous material. Fine filaments (about 20-40Å in diameter) pass through the lamina lucida, extending from the lamina densa to the basal cell membrane. These filaments are especially prominent at the sites of the hemidesmosomes, which will be described in conjunction with the basal cell. At these sites the lamina densa appears to be slightly thickened. Anchoring fibrils, measuring about 200Å in diameter, are observed extending perpendicular to the basement membrane immediately adjacent to it at its connective tissue side.

Figure 11. See illustration on opposite page.

A. Basement lamina region of clinically normal human attached gingiva. The basal lamina (b) closely follows the contour of the plasmalemma of the basal cell and is separated from the cell membrane by the lamina lucida (1). Occasional anchoring fibrils (a) are seen at the connective tissue side of the lamina densa. The dense areas at the cell membrane are hemidesmosomes (h). Smooth-walled vesicles are noted at the cell membrane adjacent to the basal lamina. Note the abundance of tonofilaments (t), mitochondria (m), and free ribosomes (r) in the basal cell. (30,000 ×).

The most prominent elements of the connective tissue (lamina propria) of normal gingiva are fibroblasts and collagen fibrils (Fig. 11B). Fibroblasts appear as irregular, elongated cells with flattened, indented nuclei and abundant rough-surfaced endoplasmic reticulum. Bundles of collagen fibrils course through the connective tissue in random fashion. Individual collagen fibrils measure 300-500Å in diameter and exhibit typical periodic banding.

B. Lamina propria of clinically normal human gingiva. Note two fibroblasts containing large, irregular, elongated nuclei (n) and rough-surfaced endoplasmic reticulum. Bundles of collagen fibrils can be seen cut in longitudinal (1) and cross section (c). (15,000 ×).

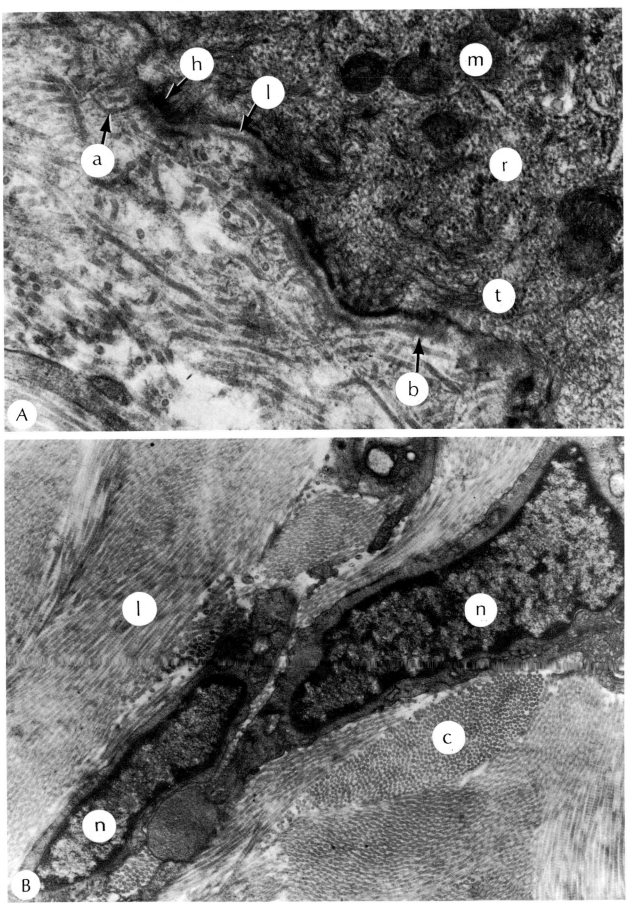

Figure 11

ELECTRON MICROSCOPY—NORMAL AND INFLAMED GINGIVA

The basal lamina shows changes in chronic inflammation (Fig. 12A). In some areas it appears thickened and diffuse, while in other areas it appears broken or absent. Such breaks in the basal lamina may provide direct communications between the connective tissue and the intercellular spaces of the epithelium.

The most prominent alterations in the normal architecture occur in the lamina propria of chronically inflamed gingiva. There appears to be a relative decrease in the number of fibroblasts and collagen fibers, with a concomitant increase in tissue spaces due to edema (Fig. 12A) and dilatation of the blood vessels. Increased numbers of macrophages, neutrophils, mast cells and plasma cells are evident. Macrophages (Fig. 12B) are identified by their large, ovoid nucleus and dense cytoplasmic bodies (lysosomes). Neutrophils contain abundant numbers of lysosomal granules. Plasma cells contain abundant rough-surfaced endoplasmic reticulum and an eccentrically placed nucleus. Mast cells exhibit cytoplasmic granules of various structure and content.

Figure 12. See illustration on opposite page.

A. In the lamina propria of chronically inflamed human gingiva large fluid containing spaces (s) replace the normally well packed collagen fibrils. The basal lamina shows both thickenings (t) and fenestrations (f). Some of these thickenings may represent preparation artefacts (compare with Fig. 11A). (35,000 ×).

B. A macrophage in the lamina propria of chronically inflamed gingiva. Note the large, oval, indented nucleus (n). The cytoplasm, in addition to containing a few cisternae of endoplasmic reticulum (e) and small vesicles, also contains lysosomes (l) of various shapes and sizes (compare with Fig. 11B). (15,000 ×).

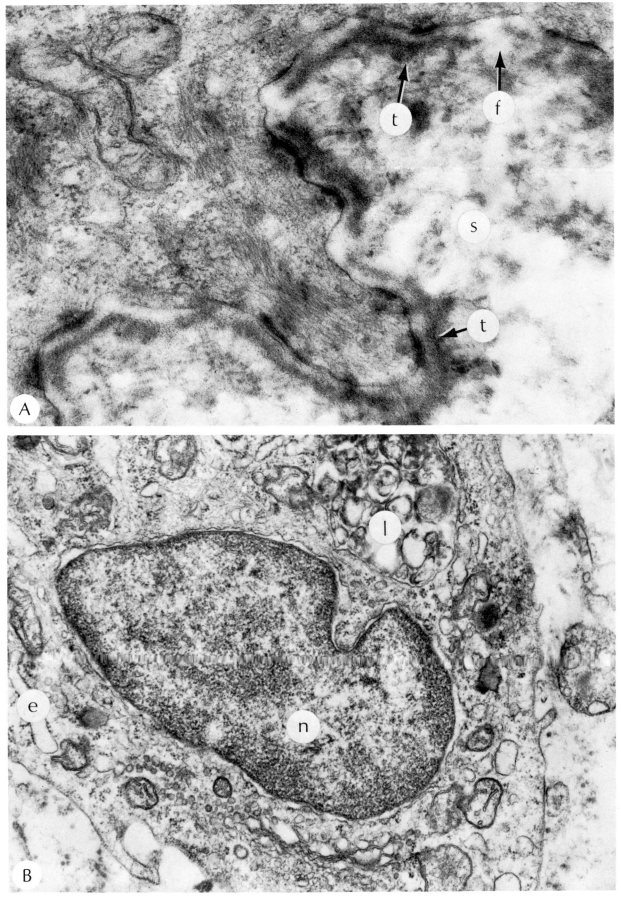

Figure 12

Plaque — Pellicle — Materia Alba

When a tooth is thoroughly cleansed and then exposed to saliva, an acellular bacterial free coating is deposited on the surface. This deposit forms in a matter of minutes, is derived from the saliva, and is called the acquired pellicle. It consists principally of glycoproteins but includes other substances such as lipids and polypeptides. Within hours, bacteria begin to deposit on the surface of the pellicle and surround themselves with a matrix which differs from that of the acquired pellicle. This aggregation of bacteria and its surrounding matrix comprise the dental plaque.

Plaque forms a soft, tenacious deposit on the surface of the tooth. It consists mainly of living and dead bacteria with a few desquamated epithelial cells and leukocytes enmeshed in a sticky protein-carbohydrate-lipid matrix. It is found throughout the mouth, mainly on the cervical third of the teeth, with the greatest accumulations occurring in the posterior areas. Lesser amounts are found on the palatal surfaces of the maxillary teeth because movements of the tongue contribute greatly to the cleansing of this area. Plaque is ivory to yellow in color and in small amounts difficult to visualize against the similarly colored background of the tooth unless it is disclosed by staining. The rate of formation of dental plaque is not constant. It varies from person to person and, in the same individual, may differ from tooth to tooth even varying in different areas around the same tooth. As it develops, the bacterial composition changes from a relatively simple largely facultative anaerobic population to a more complex one containing many anaerobic forms. Initially gram positive cocci and rods predominate. Within 2 to 3 days gram negative cocci and rods appear with filamentous forms occurring shortly thereafter. In about a week small numbers of spirochetes are frequently detectable. It is during this first week that the plaque develops its complex ecology. Later changes are more quantitative than qualitative.

The bulk of the plaque, about 80 per cent, is water; the remainder is inorganic and organic solids. Plaque adheres tenaciously to the tooth and cannot be removed readily by water sprays or rinsing. To eliminate it, some form of mechanical or frictional action, such as brushing or flossing, is necessary. In this regard, it differs from materia alba which is a non-adherent, soft, white deposit on the tooth similar in composition to plaque but easily removed by rinsing. Plaque must be eliminated because it is an important etiologic factor in gingivitis and caries. Its concentration of bacteria and bacterial products create a harmful environment capable of causing destruction of both hard and soft tissues.

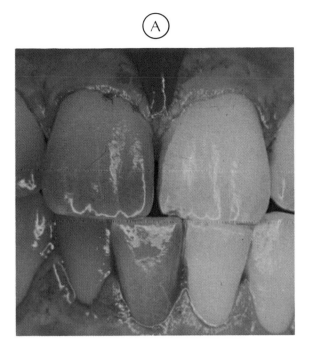

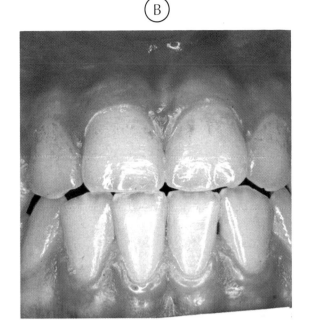

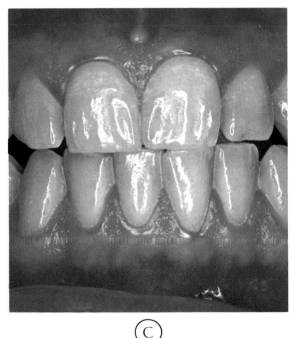

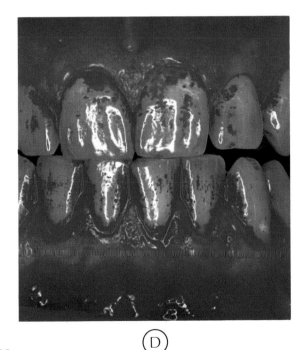

Figure 13

A. Teeth stained with basic fuchsin disclosing solution showing diffuse lightly staining pellicle. Right side cleaned with pumice to show contrast.

B. Green stain on anterior teeth of child. This discoloration is most commonly seen on the facial surfaces of the maxillary anterior teeth and occurs more frequently in boys than girls. It is generally attributed to chromogenic bacteria.

C. Anterior teeth showing three day accumulation of dental plaque.

D. Same individual as in (C) after staining with basic fuchsin disclosing solution. Note concentration of plaque interproximally and on gingival third of teeth.

CALCULUS

Calculus, sometimes called tartar, is a mineralized mass which forms on the surface of the tooth and is adherent to it. It begins as a soft bacterial laden plaque which undergoes progressive mineralization. Deposition of calculus generally begins after puberty and its prevalence increases with advancing years until age 40 when the incidence reaches about 100 per cent. Although not common, calculus may be found in very young children. Small quantities of calcified, calculus-like, material are found in germ free animals indicating that bacteria are not necessary for the process of mineralization. However, in calculus as it is found in humans, microorganisms play a prominent role in its formation. The microorganisms grow in colonies and vary according to the age of the deposit. In the first few days, cocci and rods are the prevalent organisms but in about a week filamentous forms increase in number. The time required for mineralization varies from person to person and even in the same individual there is variation around different teeth. It may begin as early as 24 to 48 hours after the initial deposition of plaque or may take two weeks or more to occur. The earliest mineralization occurs in discrete foci along the inner surface of the plaque. The foci enlarge by growth and coalescence until at maturity most of the plaque has become mineralized. However, plaque is continuously forming and is always found on the surface of the calculus.

The chemical composition of calculus is somewhat variable depending upon the age of the deposit and location from where it is taken. The differences may depend on the composition of the saliva and gingival fluid in the area where the mineralization occurred. In general, calculus consists of about 70 to 90 per cent inorganic material with the remainder being organic substances and water. The major inorganic constituent is calcium phosphate with the most common crystalline form being hydroxyapatite. Other compounds found in lesser amounts are calcium carbonate and magnesium phosphate. The organic components of calculus consist of carbohydrate-protein-lipid complexes, leukocytes, desquamated epithelial cells and bacteria.

Calculus may be classified according to its positional relationship to the gingiva. Supragingival calculus is found above the gingival margin and is visible on the tooth. Subgingival calculus is found below the margin of the gingiva and is hidden from view. There are some differences between these two types. The supragingival calculus is ivory to yellow in color, somewhat crumbly in consistency and relatively easily removed from the surface of the tooth with a scaler. Frequently, it is stained. It is found most often and in the greatest amounts on the lingual of the lower anterior teeth opposite the submandibular (Wharton's) duct and on the buccal of the maxillary molars opposite the opening of the parotid (Stenson's) duct. Subgingival calculus is usually dark in color, brown or black; dense, hard and flint-like in consistency and flattened. It adheres tenaciously to the tooth and is more difficult to remove than supragingival calculus. The current opinion is that supragingival calculus sometimes called salivary calculus derives its minerals from the saliva and subgingival calculus sometimes termed serumal calculus derives them from the gingival fluid.

Calculus, with its ever present associated covering of soft bacterial plaque, is a significant local irritant and plays an important role in the pathogenesis of periodontal disease.

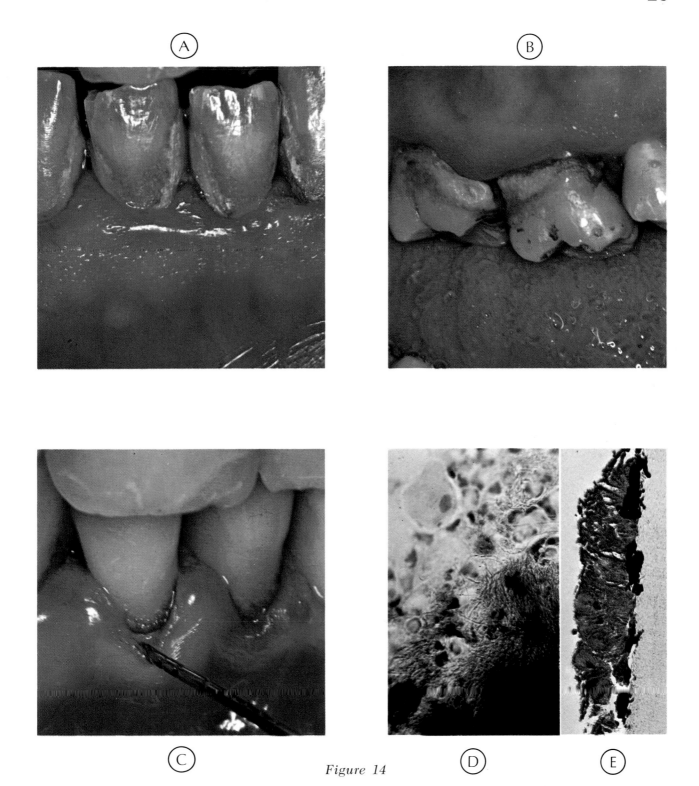

Figure 14

A & B. Supragingival calculus on facial of mandibular anterior teeth (A) and palatal of maxillary molar teeth (B). Note yellowish, crumbly, clay-like appearance.

C. Dense, brown subgingival calculus disclosed by deflecting the tissue with a probe. Note inflamed swollen gingiva.

D. Smear of calculus and plaque showing deeply staining bacteria (mainly filamentous). Note desquamated epithelial cell containing nucleus (upper left) and numerous adjacent leukocytes.

E. Plaque stained with von Kossa silver technic showing early calculus formation. The darkly staining foci on the surface (right) are areas of calcification. Filamentous bacteria predominate but rod and coccal forms are also present.

INTERDENTAL (COL) AREA

The interdental (interproximal) space beneath the contact area of adjacent teeth is called the gingival embrasure. This space is occupied by the interdental gingiva (gingival papilla). When viewed buccally or lingually the interdental gingiva is triangular in shape with the apex pointed occlusally. The size and shape of the interdental papilla is dependent upon the size and shape of its embrasure. Between the buccal and lingual triangular peaks of tissue there is a valley-like depression known as the col. If, instead of being in contact, there are spaces or diastemas between the teeth, the gingival embrasures are missing. In that event, the interdental gingiva does not have the characteristic triangular shape with buccal and lingual peaks of tissue and an intervening col area. The interdental papilla is lacking and the tissue tightly bound down to the alveolus.

As the tooth erupts, the tissue lining the col is composed of non-keratinized odontogenic (dental) epithelium. However, the facial and lingual surfaces of the interdental gingiva are covered with stratified squamous oral epithelium which is either keratinized or parakeratinized. During the process of eruption and for a time thereafter, epithelial cells which appear to be odontogenic are still recognizable in the col area. The tissue in this region is similar to that of the epithelial attachment since both are derived from the reduced enamel epithelium. In both instances, the odontogenic epithelium is gradually undermined and replaced by non-keratinized stratified squamous oral epithelium which is devoid of rete ridges. Some investigators suggest that during the period of replacement the col is an area of weakness as it is protected only by a thin covering of odontogenic epithelium. They reason that this thin covering is more susceptible to injury than the somewhat thicker stratified squamous oral epithelium which gradually replaces it. Other investigators suggest that the odontogenic epithelium may not be an area of weakness. They point to the fact that there is proliferative activity in the outer layers of this type of epithelium and it is unwise to consider it degenerative. They postulate that the inflammation seen in conjunction with the dental epithelium may be due to a non-bacterial induced inflammatory response resulting from compression and breakdown of the connective tissue about the erupting tooth and not from a defective epithelial covering.

In the underlying connective tissue of the col, bands of collagen fibers cover the alveolar bone and form a fibrous attachment to it. Other collagen fiber bundles extend bucco-lingually into the peaks of the papillae forming the main bulk of the tissue in these areas. Blood vessels, lymphatics and nerves are found in the less dense surrounding interstitial connective tissue.

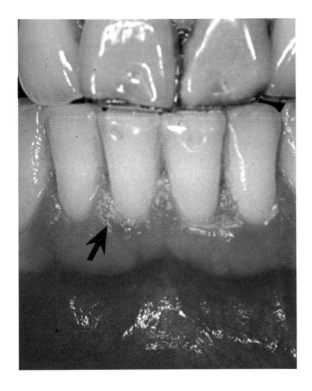

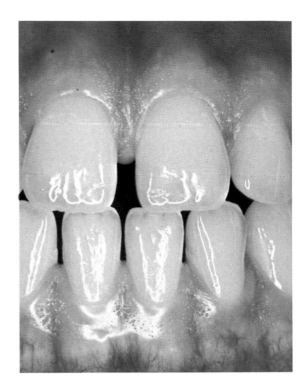

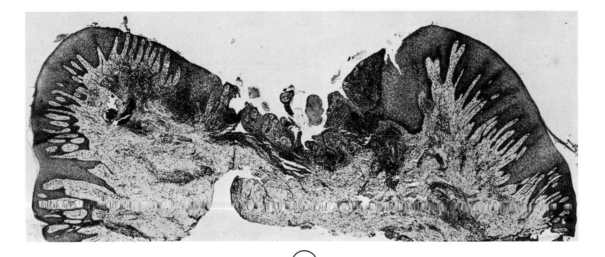

Figure 15

A. Interproximal (interdental) gingiva in mandibular anterior region showing embrasures with triangular shaped papillae. Arrow indicates area from which tissue seen in (C) was obtained.

B. Anterior region showing spaces (diastemas) of varying size between the teeth. Note flattened interdental papillae and absence of col in these areas.

C. Tissue section taken from interdental area indicated by arrow in (A) showing buccal (left) and lingual (right) peaks and intervening col. Note severe inflammatory reaction with ulceration and necrosis of tissue in the col area. The inflammation has spread buccally and lingually, causing proliferation and degeneration in both epithelium and connective tissue. The clinical appearance (A, arrow) shows only slight inflammatory involvement.

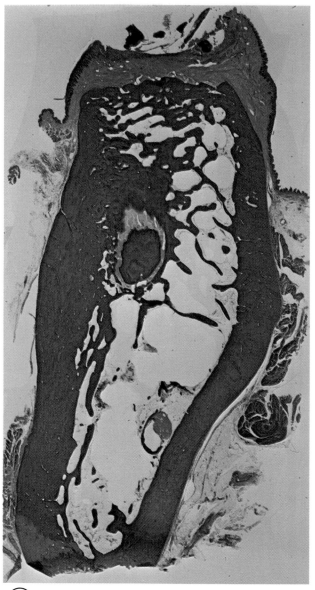

(A)

Figure 16

A. Section of mandible showing interdental region between second and third molars. The solid oval structure surrounded by connective tissue (periodontal ligament) seen in the central area of the jaw is a portion of a root. Below and to the right of this area is a circular ring of bone, the mandibular canal, which contains blood vessels and nerves.

Figure 16B and C.   See illustrations on opposite page.

B. Interdental region shown in Fig. 16A with buccal gingival peak (right), lingual gingival peak (left) and depressed central col area joining them. The epithelium lining the col is hyperplastic in some areas and thinned and ulcerated in others.

C. High power of col area and peak of buccal gingival papilla shown in Fig. 16B. There is considerable debris present and bacterial colonization is noted in this region. The underlying connective tissue is densely infiltrated with inflammatory cells and devoid of epithelial covering. Numerous dilated blood vessels are present. In an area such as this, bleeding may occur spontaneously.

Interdental (Col) Area

Access for adequate cleansing in the interdental col area is a problem for many patients. The anatomy of this region makes removal of local irritants from the depressed central area extremely difficult. As a result, this portion of the col is usually the most inflamed. The epithelium lining the col may be hyperplastic towards the periphery but in the central area it is generally atrophic and ulcerated. Exposure of the underlying connective tissue to the oral fluids results in a continued severe inflammatory response. There is a dense infiltration with leukocytes, the majority being lymphocytes and plasma cells. The connective tissue in this area bleeds readily upon slight provocation and may bleed spontaneously, if the injured capillaries rupture. The collagen fibers are fragmented and destroyed. Much debris tends to collect and remain in this region and bacteria multiply readily in this relatively protected environment. Inflammation spreads from this area buccally and lingually and may have to reach the outer facial and lingual surfaces before the disease becomes clinically apparent. At the same time, the inflammation may be extending apically into the bone. When the interdental gingival tissue is surgically removed, it usually takes four to eight weeks for clinical healing to appear complete. The rate and thoroughness of the healing depend on how well the area is kept clean.

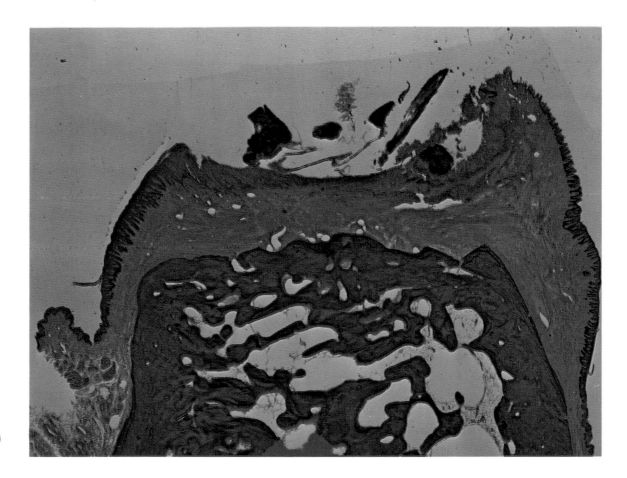

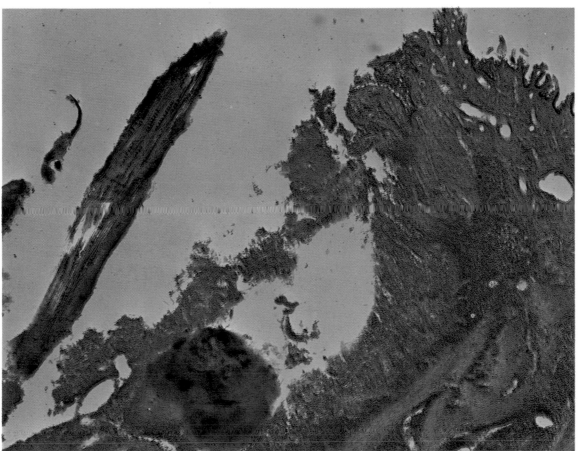

Figure 16 (Continued)

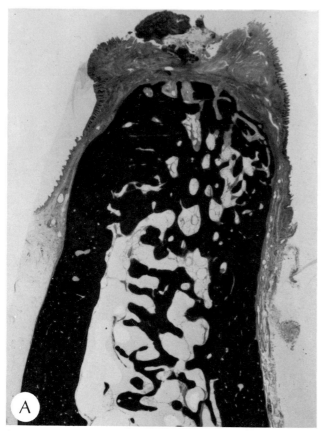

A. Bucco-lingual section of interdental area showing the col between the canine and first premolar teeth.

B. Higher power of col illustrated in (A). The gingiva is inflamed with the most severe response in the central depressed region. The epithelium is ulcerated in this area leaving a raw connective tissue surface. Some debris, both calcified and non-calcified, is present. Note bands of collagen fibers extending from buccal to lingual over the crest of the bone.

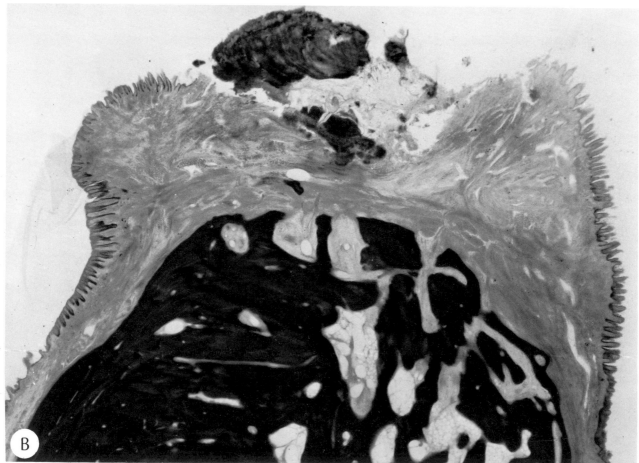

Figure 17

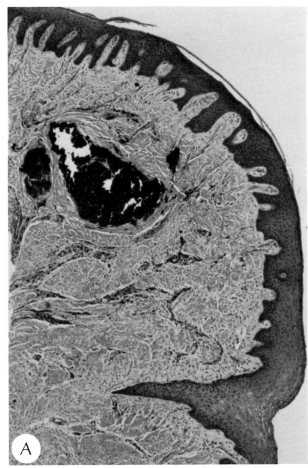

A. Gingival tissue covered with stratified squamous epithelium showing strands of keratin on the surface. There are three areas of embedded amalgam particles (black) which elicit only a mild inflammatory response. The particles are being encapsulated with connective tissue.

B. Gingival tissue containing several calcified foreign bodies. These particles are fragments of calculus which often become embedded in the gingiva and may cause a severe inflammatory reaction.

C. High power of rodent gingival connective tissue showing numerous fragments of hair-like foreign bodies. There is an intense inflammatory reaction to these particles. Large foreign body giant cells form part of the inflammatory response.

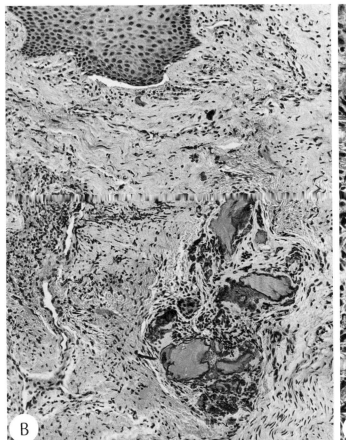

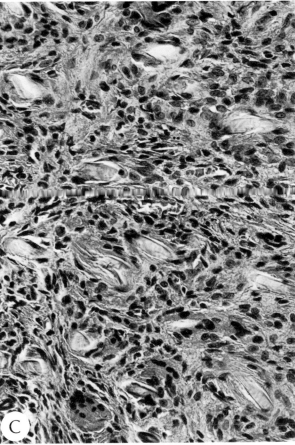

Figure 18

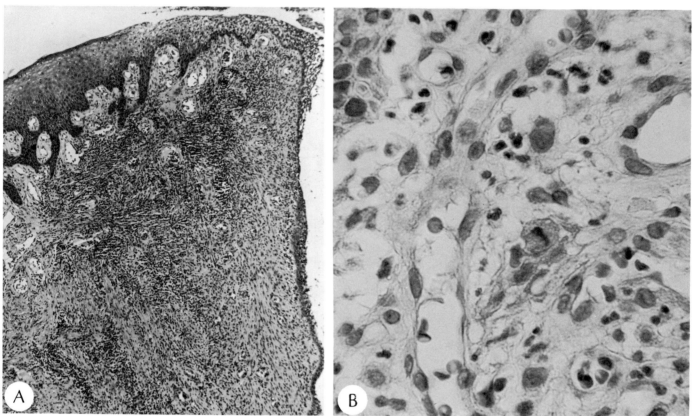

Figure 19

A. Inflamed marginal gingiva. The epithelium on the outer surface is hyperplastic. At the tip of the crest, the epithelium is degenerating and the lateral wall of the pocket (right) is lined with a thin layer of epithelium which, in some areas, is ulcerated. The connective tissue is densely infiltrated with inflammatory cells. Numerous dilated blood vessels are present, particularly in the papillary connective tissue.

B. Higher power of inflamed gingival tissue seen in (A). The connective tissue is loose and edematous. There are many dilated capillaries, some of which contain blood cells. The tissue is infiltrated with inflammatory cells.

GINGIVA — INFLAMMATORY CELLS

The majority of the inflammatory cells found in chronic marginal gingivitis are lymphocytes and plasma cells. Other cell types seen in lesser number are histiocytes (macrophages), polymorphonuclear leukocytes and mast cells.

Lymphocytes vary in diameter from eight to ten microns. The nucleus is relatively large, darkly staining and is surrounded by a narrow band of cytoplasm which stains pale blue. Often the cytoplasm is not visible and the lymphocyte appears as a round mass of chromatin. These cells are seen after the polymorphonuclear leukocytes in the inflammatory process and are characteristic of chronic inflammation. Lymphocytes possess random motility, are mildly phagocytic and may neutralize injurious products of a bacterial nature. There is some question as to whether they produce antibodies or simply transport them to the injured area.

Plasma cells are oval, 10 to 12 microns in diameter and contain an eccentrically placed nucleus in a basophilic cytoplasm. Bits of chromatin are dispersed at the periphery of the cell creating a "cartwheel" appearance. It is thought that they are derived from immature lymphoid type cells. Plasma cells are found in the tissues but are not normally present in the circulating blood. They appear late (after four to five days) in the inflammatory process and are usually mixed with lymphocytes. Plasma cells are found in greater proportion in inflammatory reactions in the gingiva than in other areas of the body. This has given rise to the theory that gingival inflammation may, in part, be an antigen-antibody reaction as plasma cells contain high concentrations of gamma globulin and are thought to be the primary source of antibody synthesis.

Histiocytes (macrophages) are large phagocytic cells about 15 to 20 microns in diameter. They are motile, move in an ameboid manner and remove debris and bacteria in the inflamed area. They are derived from primitive mesenchymal tissue particularly of the reticulo-endothelial system.

(Text continued on page 34)

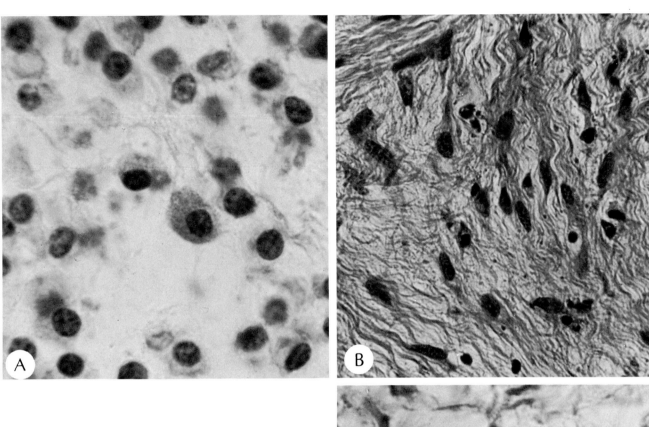

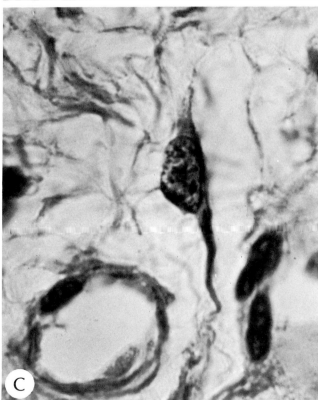

A. Cellular phase of inflammatory process. The majority of the inflammatory cells contain cartwheel nuclei characteristic of plasma cells. A mast cell with coarse granular basophilic cytoplasm is present in the center of the field. Above and to the right of the mast cell at the edge of the field is a large macrophage.

B. Newly forming connective tissue. Numerous plump fibroblastic nuclei with spindle-shaped projecting cytoplasm are present. There are strands of collagen fibrils combining to form larger bundles. Interspersed among the fibroblasts are small lymphocytes.

C. Early stage of connective tissue formation. The tissue is edematous and contains numerous strands of fibrillar connective tissue. A large, plump, young fibroblast is noted in the center of the field. A newly formed capillary with prominent endothelial cells is seen below and to the left.

Figure 20

GINGIVA — INFLAMMATORY CELLS (*Continued*)

Polymorphonuclear leukocytes are found early in the inflammatory process usually within the first hours of injury. These cells contain lysosomes which are known to be capable of releasing more than two dozen digestive enzymes. They are derived from bone marrow, carried in the blood, and released by the injured vessels. The nucleus of the mature cell is segmented and is composed of two to five lobes. Polymorphonuclear leukocytes are similar in size to plasma cells, i.e., 10 to 12 microns in diameter and are motile, ameboid and phagocytic. They are the first and most numerous cell to be found in the acute phase of the inflammatory reaction. If the inflammatory reaction continues as in chronic marginal gingivitis, these cells diminish in number while the lymphocytes, plasma cells and histiocytes increase.

Mast cells contain coarse cytoplasmic granules which stain metachromatically. These cells carry or produce many substances such as histamine and heparin. It is probable that most of these active compounds are located within the cytoplasmic granules. Mast cells are located about small blood vessels and are capable of releasing substances into the blood stream as well as into the surrounding connective tissue. They are active early in the inflammatory process. It is thought that the inflammatory stimulus causes degranulation of these cells resulting in fewer mast cells in areas of severe inflammation than in areas of slight inflammation or in normal tissues.

INTERDENTAL PAPILLA — INFLAMMATION

Careful examination of the interdental papilla is of paramount importance as it is in this region that some of the earliest clinical signs of gingival disease occur. Variations from the normal in color, size, shape, texture and consistency as well as bleeding tendencies are included in the changes. The initial lesion develops in the col or at the base of the sulcus but in either case, the pathology is usually reflected in the interdental area. The incidence of gingivitis in this region is greater than in other areas of the mouth because the anatomic relationships permit the accumulation and retention of local irritants and make cleansing difficult.

The introduction of an irritant into the interdental area results in an inflammatory response. The appearance of inflammatory cells in the connective tissue is associated with vascular changes which cause alterations in color, size, shape, texture and consistency. There is proliferation and degeneration of the epithelium and connective tissue and disruption of the basal lamina. The earliest changes in the inflammatory response are vascular in nature. There are many thin-walled, dilated, engorged blood vessels and an increased number of capillaries, many of which become thrombosed. The connective tissue of the papilla becomes edematous and heavily infiltrated with leukocytes resulting in destruction and fragmentation of the collagen fibers. The most common inflammatory cells are lymphocytes and plasma cells. Macrophages are present in relation to the necrotic material and tissue debris. In some instances, pus is a clinical finding. This is a thick, yellowish-white liquid composed principally of bacteria, necrotic leukocytes and tissue debris all undergoing proteolytic digestion. Bleeding into the tissues as a result of necrosis of capillary walls is a common finding. This may occur spontaneously or from slight pressure on the tissue.

Changes in the epithelium take place coincident with the destruction of the underlying connective tissue. The basal lamina may break down, removing the barrier to direct invasion of the epithelium by the migrating inflammatory cells. The epithelial cells begin to proliferate and penetrate into the connective tissue. This proliferating epithelium may appear microscopically as cords, nests or loops of cells. The normal basal cells are cuboidal with large round nuclei and relatively little cytoplasm. The proliferating cells are smaller and stain more deeply. There may be intra and extracellular edema of the basal and prickle cell layers with the epithelium becoming edematous (spongiotic). Necrosis of the epithelium may occur resulting in areas of ulceration with exposure of the underlying connective tissue.

The inflammatory reaction is essentially a healing process. It is the method by which the body repairs and heals itself. In the normal course of events, when the irritant or initiator of the inflammation is removed, the proliferative phase of the inflammatory response predominates and the degenerating and necrotic tissue is removed and repaired. The inflammatory reaction then goes on to completion and the lesion is healed. If the local irritant causing the inflammation is not removed, the lesion remains. Complete healing cannot take place and the result is continued destruction of the tissues with eventual loss of the tooth.

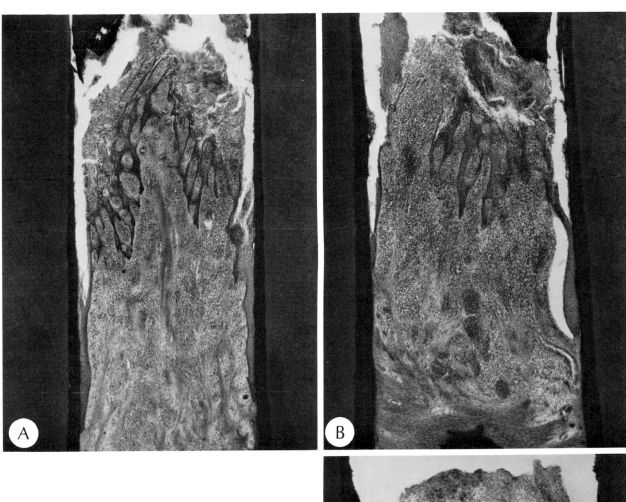

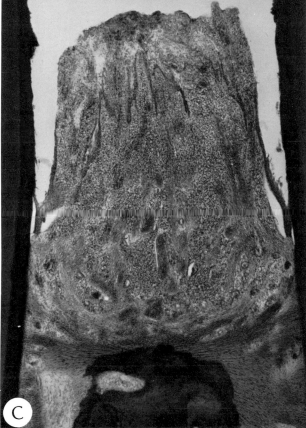

A. Interdental papilla showing infiltration with leukocytes and degeneration of connective tissue. Note proliferation of epithelium in the crestal region in an attempt to wall off the necrotic tissue on the surface. Note, too, the proliferation of the epithelial attachment along the root.

B. Inflamed interdental papilla. The crest of the papilla on the left is ulcerated; on the right, proliferating epithelium undermines the necrotic tissue. Note impingement of calculus (top right) on the crest of the papilla.

C. Inflamed interdental papilla. The gingival fibers are fragmented and destroyed by the leukocytic infiltrate but in spite of the severe inflammatory response many of the transseptal fibers covering the bone remain intact.

Figure 21

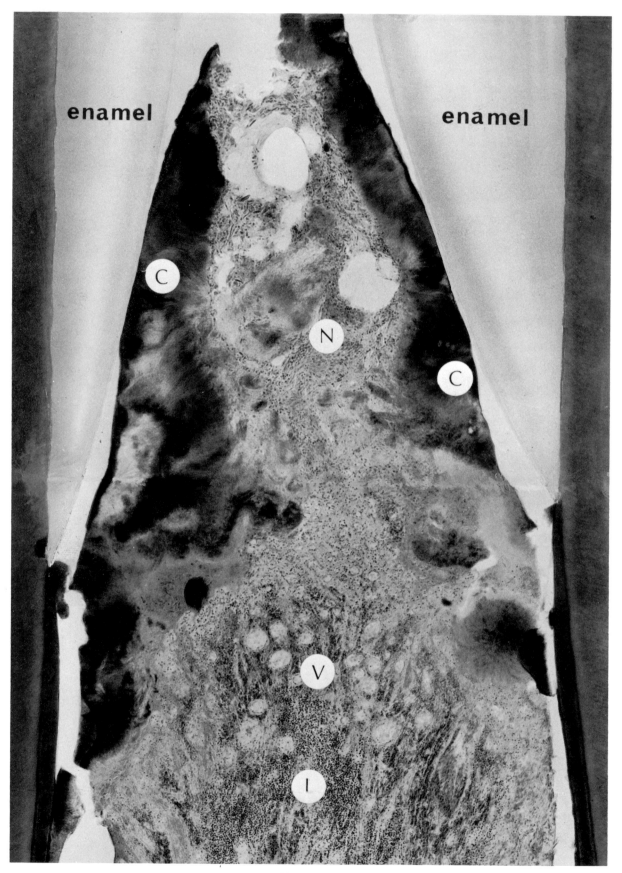

Figure 22

Mesio-distal section of interdental papilla. Calculus (C) is present on both tooth surfaces. The central portion of the papilla is composed of necrotic tissue (N) and debris. There are numerous capillaries (V) surrounded by a dense inflammatory infiltrate (L) which has fragmented and destroyed the collagen fibers. Note: Enamel dissolved in tissue preparation has been replaced by drawing to show relationship of papilla to teeth.

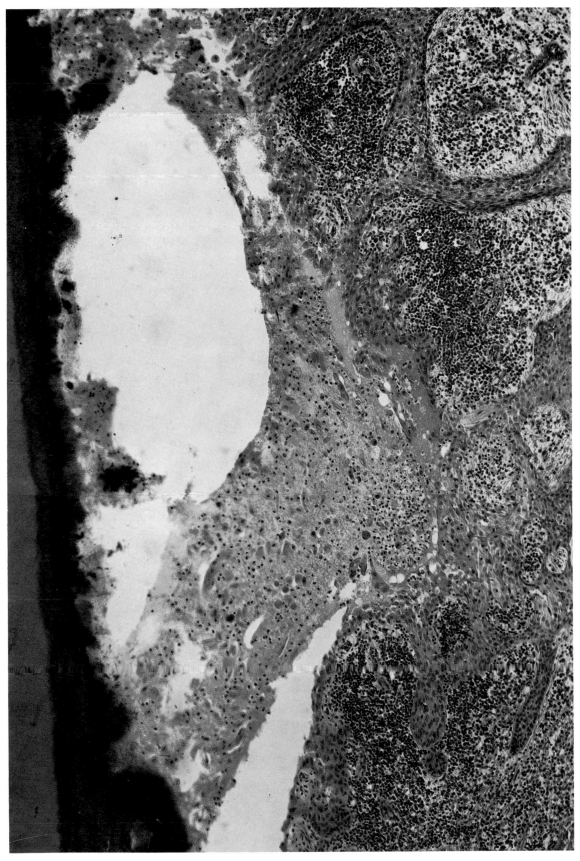

Figure 23

High power of pocket area showing portion of tooth (left) and interdental papilla (right). The tooth surface is covered with calculus and bacteria. There is a very dense leukocytic infiltrate in the papilla. The epithelium is proliferating in some areas and is degenerating and necrotic in others. A considerable amount of intra and extracellular edema is present. Note the large area of necrotic tissue, bacteria and debris extending from the papilla to the tooth. Clinically, this would be expressed as pus.

GINGIVA — CHILDREN

There are slight variations in the normal gingival and periodontal tissues of the child when compared with those of an adult. In the child the gingival epithelium is thinner, less keratinized and more vascular. For these reasons it appears more red. The gingiva of the child is less fibrous because of the decreased density of connective tissue fibers in the lamina propria and as a result is softer than that of the adult. The gingival margin is often blunted or thickened owing to the inflammation and resultant hyperemia and edema that accompanies eruption. Stippling in the child is less pronounced than in the adult and is sometimes absent. The cementum is generally thinner and the periodontal ligament is usually wider with fewer fibers, less dense fiber bundles and increased vascular supply. The alveolar bone often has larger marrow spaces, fewer trabeculae and a thinner lamina dura.

Chronic marginal gingivitis is the most prevalent gingival disease in children. The gingiva presents all the changes in color, size, shape and consistency and texture characteristically seen in adults with this condition. Epidemiological studies of children ranging in age from one to eighteen years from different parts of the world and from varying racial, social, and economic backgrounds, have shown that 60 to 90 per cent presented with at least some degree of gingivitis.

Periodontitis occurs when the inflammation from the gingiva has extended into the underlying periodontal structures. Although gingival inflammation is a frequent finding in children, periodontitis is uncommon. In those cases that have been reported there is marked alveolar bone resorption with periodontal pocket formation.

Acute herpetic gingivostomatitis is the most common acute gingival infection of childhood. It is caused by the Herpes simplex virus. It is commonly seen in children between the ages of two and six but may also be found in adolescents and young adults. (Described on page 72.)

Thrush (Moniliasis) is a fungal infection whose etiologic agent is Candida (Monilia) albicans. It is found in infants, the elderly, and debilitated patients. (Described on page 72.)

Acute necrotizing ulcerative gingivitis (Vincent's infection) is rare in children. However, it has been reported to occur following acute inflammatory and other debilitating diseases. The child often has a fever with general discomfort and lymphadenopathy. (Described on page 54.)

Papillon-Lefevre is an extremely rare syndrome which affects the periodontium of young children. The deciduous teeth erupt at the normal time. However, they soon become loose as a result of alveolar bone loss. There is severe gingival inflammation with periodontal pockets. The children are usually uncomfortable and frequently all the primary teeth have to be extracted or are exfoliated at an early age. Longer term studies of these children indicate that the permanent dentition is also involved. The permanent teeth erupt normally but because of the rapid periodontal destruction, these teeth are lost within two to three years. These patients are often edentulous by 12 to 15 years of age. The third molars are also lost within a few years after eruption. In addition to the oral problems there is hyperkeratosis of the palms of the hands and soles of the feet. The etiology of this syndrome is not known. Affected children that display a familial disposition for this condition show an autosomal recessive mode of inheritance.

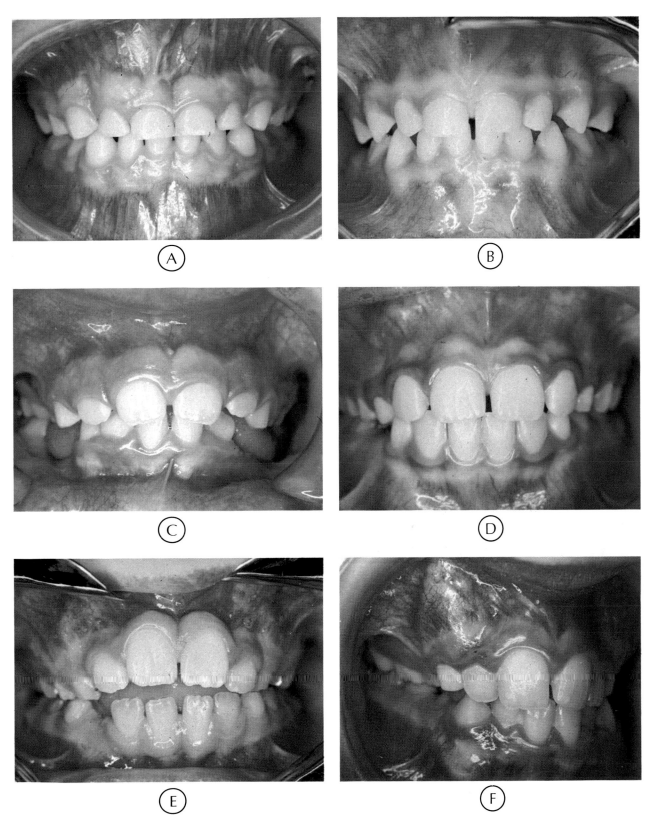

Figure 24

A. Primary dentition in a three-year-old child with marginal inflammation. (B) shows a three-year-old child with brownish-yellow gingival pigmentation. (C-F) show seven to nine-year-old children with mixed dentitions and gingivitis. There is melanin pigmentation of the gingiva in the child illustrated in (D) (compare with (B)). Note that gingivitis increases in severity during periods of tooth eruption and when local irritants accumulate.

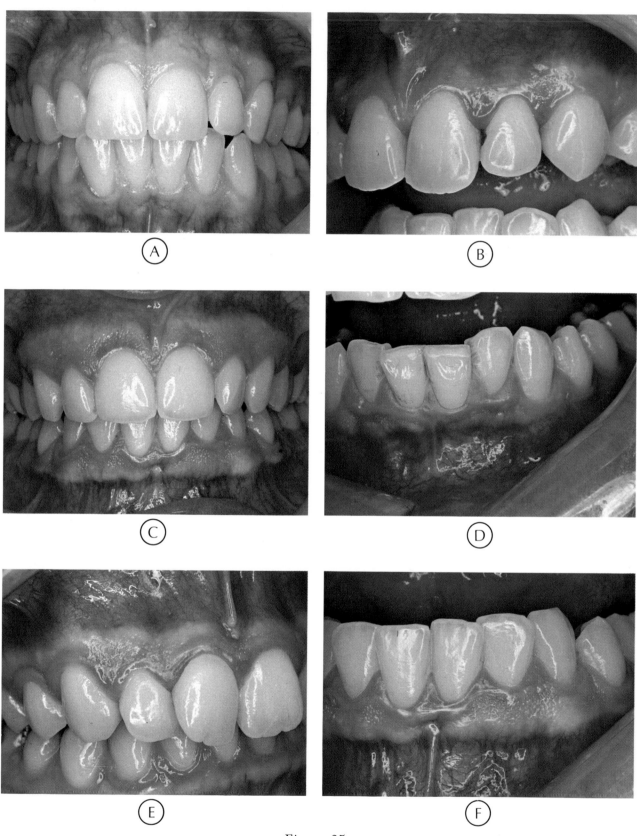

Figure 25

Early stages of chronic marginal gingivitis. (A) shows very slight marginal redness and slight swelling of the papillae, particularly in the mandibular anterior region. In (B) there is pronounced enlargement and redness between the central and lateral incisors associated with caries. (C-F) show marginal and papillary inflammation. Note that as the swelling becomes more pronounced the stippling tends to disappear.

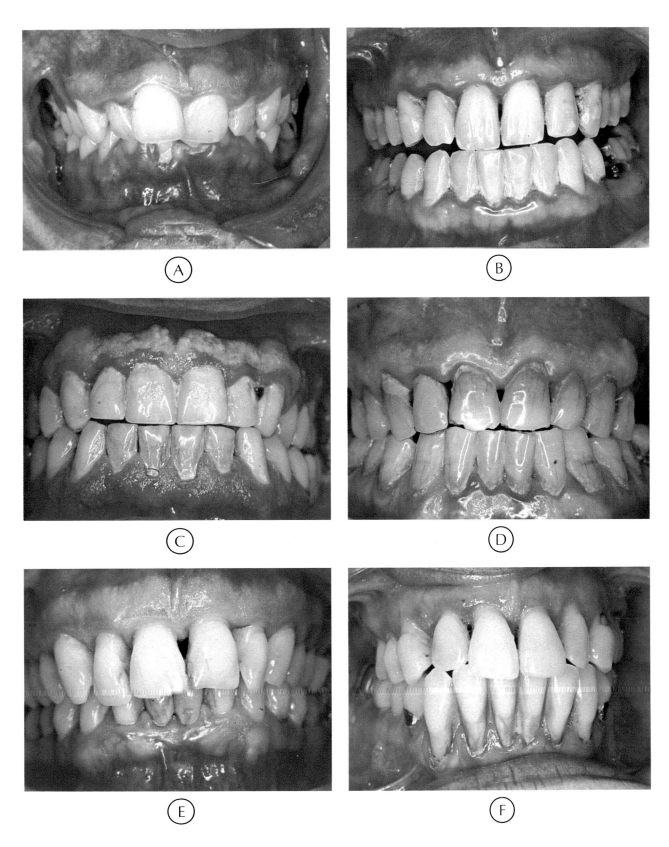

Figure 26

   Gingival recession may be categorized two ways: (a) observable clinically, and (b) hidden by gingiva. Hidden recession is measured by inserting a probe to the level of the epithelial attachment. The former (a) is the apparent position of the gingiva and the latter (b) the actual position. It is the actual or probed position which determines the severity of the recession. (A-F) show the apparent (unprobed) gingival position.

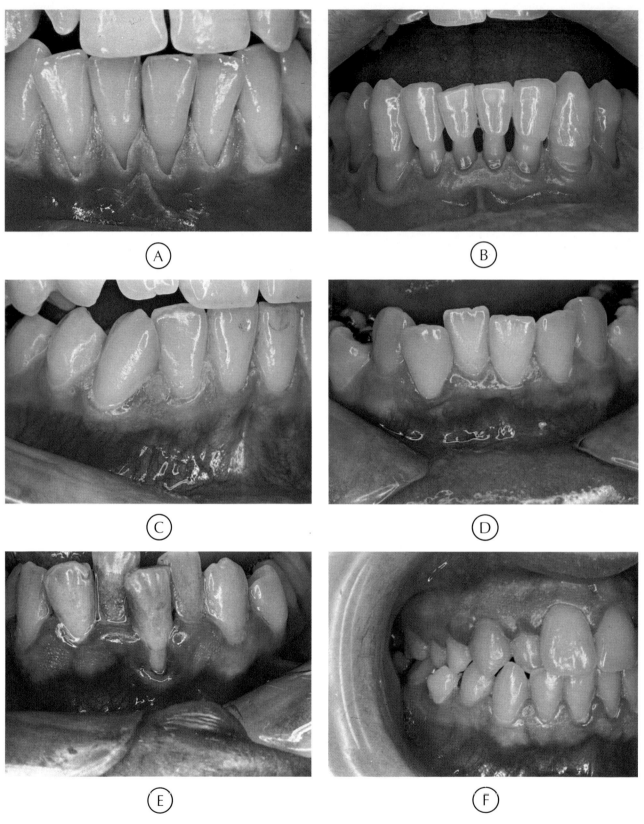

Figure 27

(A) "V"-shaped clefting and recession of the gingiva in the mandibular incisor teeth. (B) Severe recession with abrasion. The hard enamel surface is not abraded as readily as the softer root, thus allowing the crown to stand out sharply. (C-F) Malposed teeth resulting in enlarged papillae owing to poor anatomic relationships and difficulty in cleansing. Note in (E) prominent labial version of central incisor combined with local irritation has resulted in severe localized recession with loss of attached gingiva.

GINGIVAL RECESSION—CLEFTS AND FESTOONS

Recession is defined as progressive exposure of the root surface caused by apical migration of the epithelial attachment and gingiva. It is a term that relates to the position of the gingiva on the tooth, not to the health of the tissue, which may be either normal or diseased. Concurrent with this apical shift in gingival position is loss of supporting alveolar bone and periodontal ligament. Gingival recession is found at all ages but its incidence and severity increase with age. When similar groups are compared, men have more recession than women. About 50 per cent of individuals show some degree of recession by age 25 and by age 50 almost everyone has recession. The greatest increase in recession is seen in the third through fifth decades. Recession may be localized to just one or a few teeth or it may be generalized around many teeth. It is more common on the facial than the lingual or palatal surfaces, particularly in the maxillary canine and premolar areas. Less frequently, it may be found on the lingual surfaces of the mandibular molars and incisors. Gingival recession will result in enlarged interproximal spaces which may act as food traps and on occasion may also reduce or eliminate the attached gingiva creating mucogingival problems. In addition, many people are concerned about esthetics, particularly in the anterior region and they find the increased visible root surface unattractive.

The concept of continuous physiologic eruption postulates an apical migration of the epithelial attachment and gingiva along the tooth surface with simultaneous reduction in height of the alveolar bone. Concurrent with this apical migration, there is continuous deposition of cementum and eruption of the tooth with compensatory attrition of the occlusal surface. The normal position of the gingiva varies with age. In the young, the epithelial attachment is on the enamel. In the old, it is on the root surface. Some people question the idea of continuous eruption and consider any migration of the epithelial attachment apical to the cemento-enamel junction as pathologic. The prevalent opinion accepts the former concept and considers a small amount of recession (root exposure) a normal process of aging.

There are many factors to consider in the etiology of pathologic gingival recession, such as improper position of the tooth in the arch. If the tooth is malposed, the alveolar plate may be thinned, reduced in height or even entirely lacking. The gingiva is then attached directly to the cementum of the tooth rather than to the bone. It is postulated that the former union is weaker and permits earlier and more rapid recession. Other explanations for recession are excessive pull on the gingiva from freni (muscle attachments), improper and overly vigorous toothbrushing; overhanging margins in faulty dental restorations; poor prosthetic appliances; and trauma from occlusion.

Gingival (Stillman's) clefts are extremely narrow or slit-like grooves extending apically from the gingival margin for varying distances along the tooth surface. Stillman considered them to be due to trauma from occlusion. Other suggested etiologic factors are toothbrush injury and slits in periodontal pockets which epithelialize on both sides leaving a narrow cleft.

McCall's festoons are enlargements of the gingival margin which form a thickened collar of tissue around the tooth. They can develop in the absence of inflammation in which case the tissue is normal in color and consistency. However, they are usually secondarily inflamed. Trauma from occlusion is considered an etiologic factor but festoons occur in teeth where function is absent.

GINGIVAL ENLARGEMENT

Enlargement of the gingiva is a frequent finding in gingival disease. This increase in size usually results from a combination of factors which includes proliferation of epithelial and connective tissue cells, production of additional intercellular substances, and infiltration with fluids and leukocytes from an inflammatory process. Rarely, gingival enlargement occurs in the absence of inflammation. When this happens, the increase in size results from the first two factors. The term hypertrophic gingivitis, meant to connote gingival enlargement, should not be used. Hypertrophy means enlargement of a tissue or organ as a result of increase in size of its component cells resulting from more frequent or vigorous use. Since enlargement of the gingiva does not occur because of an increase in cell size or as a result of added function, the use of the term hypertrophy in relation to the gingiva is incorrect.

For descriptive purposes gingival enlargement may be designated according to location or distribution as follows:

Localized—Limited to the gingiva in relation to a single tooth or group of teeth.
Generalized—Involving the gingiva throughout the mouth.
Marginal—Confined to the marginal gingiva.
Papillary—Confined to the interdental papillae.
Diffuse—Involving the marginal and attached gingiva and papillae.
Discrete—An isolated sessile or pedunculated mass.

A case of gingival enlargement may then be described as localized or generalized with marginal, papillary or diffuse involvement.

Gingival enlargement may also be classified according to its etiology and histopathologic changes in the following manner:

I. Inflammatory Enlargement
    A. Chronic
        1. Localized or Generalized
        2. Discrete
    B. Acute
        1. Gingival abscess
        2. Periodontal abscess
II. Noninflammatory Hyperplastic Enlargement (gingival hyperplasia)
    A. Gingival hyperplasia associated with Dilantin therapy.
    B. Familial, hereditary or idiopathic hyperplastic gingival enlargement.
III. Combined Enlargement
    (Occurs when noninflammatory gingival hyperplasia is complicated by secondary inflammatory changes.)
IV. Conditioned Enlargement
    (Occurs when the systemic condition of the individual exaggerates or distorts the usual gingival response to local irritation.)
    A. Hormonal
        1. Enlargement of pregnancy.
        2. Enlargement of puberty.
    B. Leukemic
    C. Enlargement associated with vitamin C deficiency
    D. Nonspecific Enlargement
V. Neoplastic Enlargement
VI. Developmental Enlargement

There is nothing particularly striking or pathognomonic about the histopathologic features of chronic inflammatory gingival enlargement. It consists of an infiltration with leukocytes, predominantly lymphocytes and plasma cells, along with an increase in fluid from the injured, more permeable capillaries. The endothelial cells proliferate forming new capillaries and the existing vessels are engorged. At the same time, there is proliferation of connective tissue cells with the production of new collagen fibers and hyperplasia of the epithelium with elongation of the rete pegs. There is also degeneration of the connective tissue and epithelium resulting in ulceration and hemorrhage.

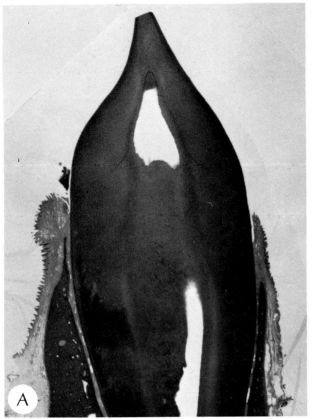

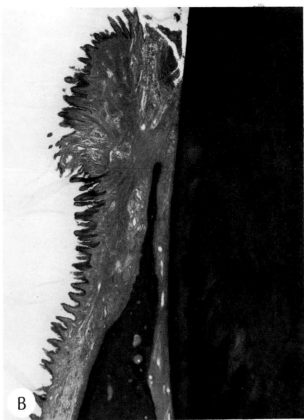

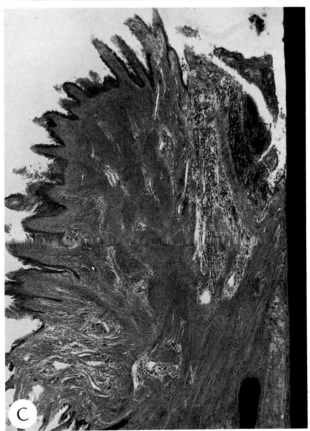

A. Bucco-lingual section of mandibular canine tooth. There is loss of alveolar bone with gingival recession.

B. Enlarged view of facial gingiva and bone shown in (A). The crestal bone is quite thin but widens considerably as it extends apically. Note dense bands of collagen fibers.

C. Higher power of facial gingiva illustrated in (A). The gingiva is enlarged and bulbous and shows a fibrotic reaction to the inflammation. Toward the facial surface (left), the collagen fibers form large bundles with leukocytes interspersed between them. In the area just beneath the pocket, the inflammation is most severe, the epithelium ulcerated, and the collagen fibers fragmented and destroyed.

Figure 28

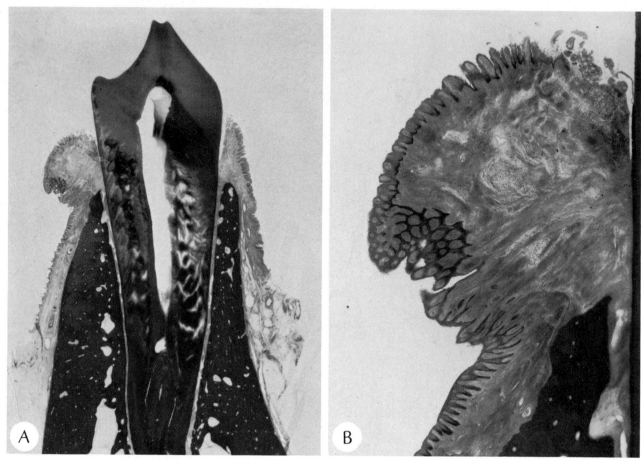

Figure 29

A, Mandibular tooth in situ. The gingiva on the lingual (right) has the normal contour while that on the buccal (left) is enlarged and bulbous. When examined in higher power (B) it can be seen that the enlarged gingiva is lined with hyperplastic stratified squamous epithelium. The epithelial hyperplasia adds to the size, but the main bulk of the enlargement comes from the connective tissue. There is a considerable amount of fibroplasia in response to the inflammation which is present not only at the base of the pocket but throughout the tissue.

GINGIVAL ENLARGEMENT

Chronic inflammation resulting from local irritation is the most common cause of gingival enlargement. Chronic inflammatory gingival enlargement may be localized to a single tooth or generalized throughout the mouth. It involves the marginal gingiva and begins as a slight swelling of the buccal and lingual tissues with a bulging of the interdental papillae. This gradually develops into a ring-like collar around the tooth which may remain relatively small or increase in size covering much of the crown of the tooth. If the enlargement is more generalized, the bulbous tissues around each tooth seem to coalesce forming a bulky undulating surface covering the entire arch. When the inflammatory response is of the edematous type, the tissues appear smooth and shiny because of the added fluid and brighter red because of the increased vascularity. The gingiva is soft, spongy, pits easily upon pressure and is not stippled. When the response to the inflammation is more proliferative, there is an increase in bulk due to fibroplasia of the connective tissue and hyperplasia of the epithelium. The tissue is pink, firm, stippled and fibrotic. The enlargement increases in size relatively slowly and, unless secondarily infected with bacteria or traumatized, is generally painless. Frequently, mouth breathers or people with open bites have enlargement of the gingiva particularly in the maxillary anterior region, as this is the area most subject to drying. Because of the greater bulk of tissue and increased pocket depth occurring in gingival enlargement, the teeth are difficult to cleanse and local irritants collect readily. As a result, ulceration, bleeding and pus formation are common clinical problems.

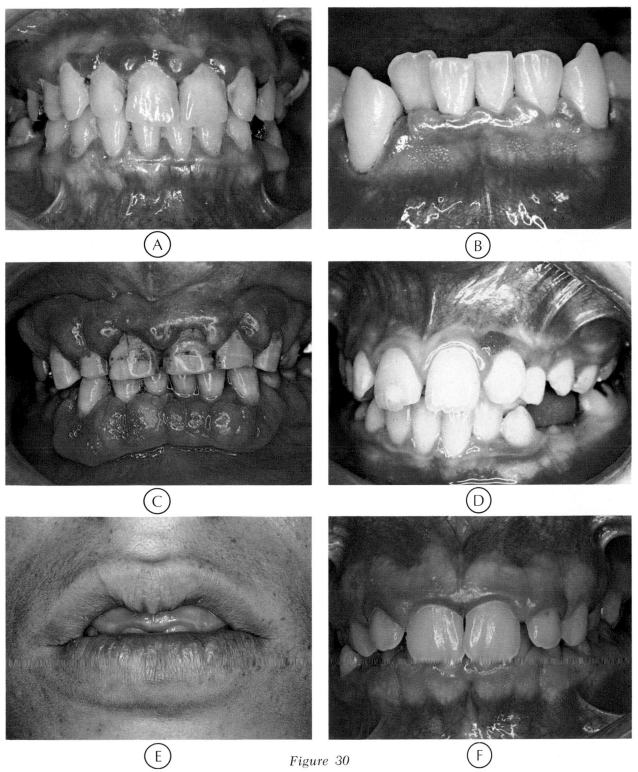

Figure 30

A. Enlarged bulbous gingiva more pronounced in the maxilla. The tissue has lost its stippling and is red, shiny and edematous.

B. Moderate gingival enlargement in the mandibular anterior region.

C. Enlarged, hyperplastic gingiva of maxilla and mandible. The tissue is more fibrotic than that seen in (A).

D. Inflamed gingiva with localized enlargement above the maxillary lateral incisor due to pyogenic granuloma.

E and F. Mouth breather showing open mouth-breathing position and enlarged, inflamed gingiva.

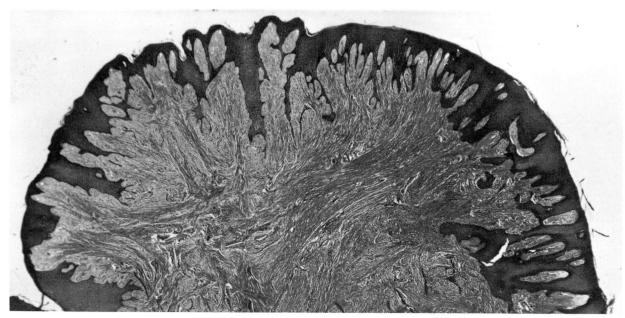

Figure 31

Enlargement of gingival tissue induced by Dilantin. The epithelium is hyperplastic and has elongated rete pegs. The underlying connective tissue is densely collagenous with large collagen fiber bundles. There is only a very slight infiltration with chronic inflammatory cells.

DILANTIN HYPERPLASIA

Dilantin (diphenylhydantoin sodium) is an anticonvulsant drug that is used in the treatment of epilepsy. It is a derivative of glycol urea and is structurally analogous to the barbiturates. It is widely used because of its effectiveness in the control and prevention of seizures and also because it is one of the few anticonvulsant drugs which does not readily oversedate the patient.

One of the distressing side reactions of medication with Dilantin is an overgrowth of the marginal gingival tissue. This does not occur in all or even a majority of the patients receiving the drug. Estimates of the incidence of gingival overgrowth vary from about three to sixty per cent with children and young adults being more commonly affected than older individuals. The basic cause for this reaction is not known. Some investigators think it is a sensitivity reaction and more especially a localized toxic reaction since this drug is found in high concentrations in the salivary glands and is excreted in the saliva.

Histologically, the lesion appears as a nonspecific hyperplasia of both epithelium and connective tissue. In the early stages, there is acanthosis of the epithelium with proliferation and deepening of the rete pegs and fibroplasia of the connective tissue with added collagen formation. Concurrently, there is an increase in blood vessels and intercellular elements. This results in a dense, firm tissue. The marked absence of inflammatory cell infiltration suggests that inflammation does not initiate the lesion but when present is a secondary complicating factor.

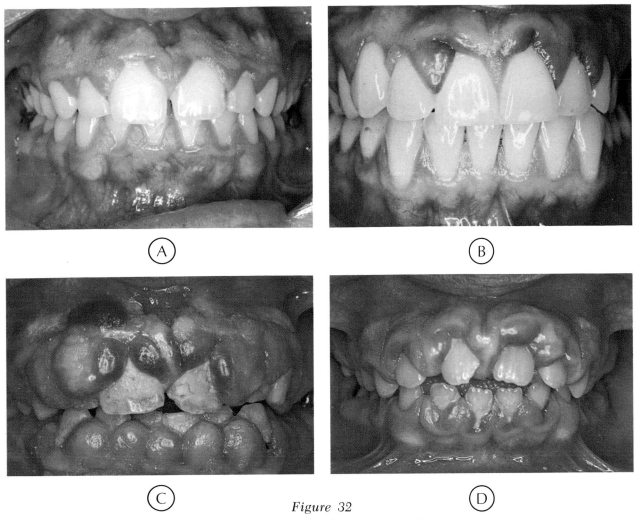

Figure 32

A and B. Early stages of Dilantin induced gingival enlargement. The hyperplasia is confined mainly to the interproximal marginal gingiva.

C and D. Advanced stages of Dilantin induced gingival enlargement. The gingiva almost covers the teeth. Note heavy deposits on the teeth.

DILANTIN HYPERPLASIA

Dilantin hyperplasia is a painless reaction unless the tissue is secondarily traumatized. The amount of overgrowth varies considerably from mouth to mouth and even varies somewhat in different areas of the same mouth. Generally, the greatest amount of hyperplasia is found on the labial of the maxillary anterior teeth. The palatal tissue is usually less involved.

Dilantin hyperplasia may occur in clinically healthy mouths with little or no evidence of inflammation. The lesion appears pink, lobulated and stippled with no tendency to bleed. It arises initially as a small overgrowth in the interproximal region and spreads buccally and lingually to form a collar or ring around the tooth. At times, the lesion may enlarge to such an extent that it almost covers the teeth. However, the size of the lesion does not appear to be related to the dosage or duration of exposure to the drug. Usually, the enlarged tissue is secondarily complicated with inflammation from local irritation. This results in a combined or additive effect with enlargement coming from both the drug and the inflammatory process. When this occurs, the tissue is softer, redder and bleeds more easily.

Hyperplasia of tissue occurs around teeth rather than in edentulous areas. Patients may have hyperplasia around teeth in one arch with no enlargement in an opposing edentulous arch. Cases have even been reported of individuals having overgrowth of tissue around abutment teeth with no overgrowth in the area of the pontic. Completely edentulous mouths are free of dilantin hyperplasia.

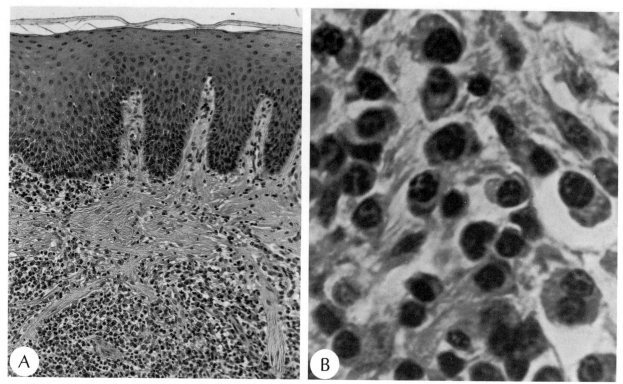

Figure 33

A. Gingival tissue from patient with acute myelogenous leukemia. There is a dense infiltration with leukemic cells. Note the papillary layer of the connective tissue just beneath the epithelium is relatively devoid of leukemic cells.

B. High power of gingival tissue showing infiltration with numerous large immature leukemic cells.

BLOOD DYSCRASIAS

Leukemia is a neoplastic blood dyscrasia involving the immature precursors of white blood cells. Oral manifestations occur frequently in both acute and subacute stages but in the chronic form there are usually no oral changes suggestive of a hematologic disturbance. In all types of leukemia local irritation is the precipitating factor for the oral changes which may be the first indication of a hematologic problem. These changes include gingival enlargement, pallor, ulceration of the mucosa, petechiae and spontaneous bleeding. The marginal and attached gingiva often appear cyanotic with a diffuse bluish-red color. The interdental papillae are blunted and edema creates a tense, smooth, shiny gingival surface with reduction or loss of stippling. The tissue is friable and bleeds on slightest provocation, often spontaneously. Hematologic changes exaggerate the response to local irritants. By removing them, it is often possible to reduce or eliminate many of the gingival changes. Leukemic enlargement does not occur in edentulous areas.

Histologically, there is a dense infiltration of immature leukemic cells in both marginal and attached gingiva. However, relatively few of these cells are found in the papillary layer of the connective tissue. This contrasts sharply with the more heavily infiltrated reticular layer. Leukemic cells fill the engorged blood vessels and also replace the normal components of the connective tissue. The epithelium may be thinned and atrophic in some areas and hyperplastic in others. Degeneration may result from inter and intracellular edema and leukocytic infiltration. The periodontal ligament and alveolar bone may also be infiltrated with leukemic cells.

Biopsies frequently show alterations in the gingiva from the leukemic process, particularly in the acute and subacute stages. However, in chronic leukemia the only apparent microscopic change may be inflammatory resulting from chronic irritation. Definitive diagnosis of all forms of leukemia is made on a hematologic basis.

Thrombocytopenic purpura is a blood dyscrasia characterized by a reduction in circulating platelets. Petechiae and hemorrhage occur spontaneously in the mouth as

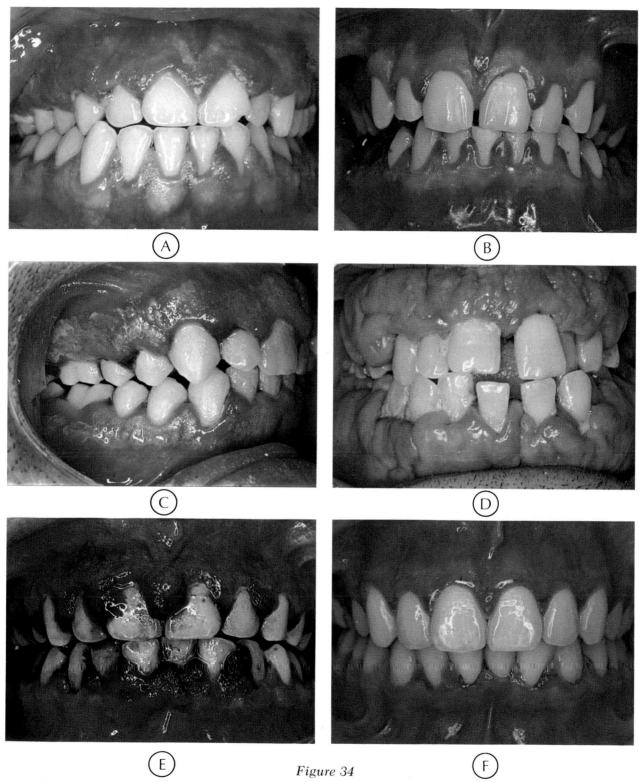

Figure 34

A-D. Leukemic enlargement of the gingiva. The gingiva often has a friable appearance with a bluish cast but varies more from individual differences than because of leukemic cell type. In (A), (B), and (D), the cell type is predominantly myelocytic; in (C), monocytic.

E and F. Idiopathic thrombocytopenic purpura. (E) shows enlarged, swollen gingiva that bleeds spontaneously. (F) The same patient after careful debridement and scaling.

well as in the skin and mucous membranes elsewhere in the body. The gingiva is edematous, swollen, soft and bleeds easily. The response to local irritation is greatly exaggerated by the hematologic problem and the elimination of all local irritants results in a dramatic change in clinical appearance.

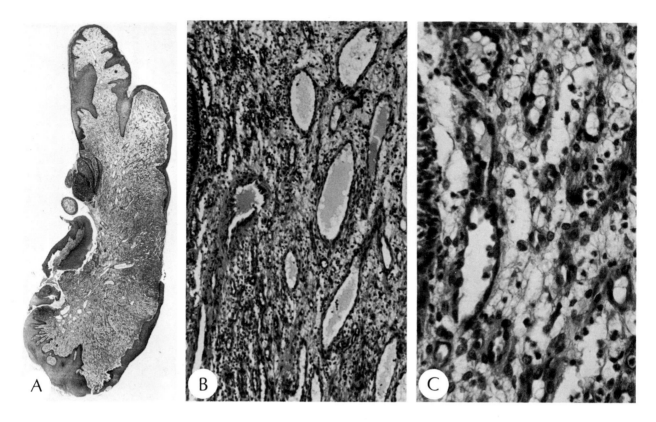

Figure 35

A. Angiogranuloma associated with pregnancy. In some areas, the epithelium is hyperplastic; in others, it is thinned, atrophic and ulcerated. The underlying connective tissue is infiltrated with inflammatory cells and contains numerous dilated vessels.

B. Higher power of connective tissue shown in A. The increased number of dilated vessels is readily apparent as is the extensive infiltrate with inflammatory cells.

C. Higher power of B. Note the edematous nature of the connective tissue. It is composed of fluid, fine fibrils, dilated vessels and inflammatory cells. There are no dense collagen bundles.

HORMONAL CHANGES

Pregnancy and puberty are normal physiologic occurrences that cause alterations in the hormonal balance. These hormonal changes exaggerate the response of the gingiva to local irritants resulting in redness, swelling, increased gingival exudate, and bleeding beyond that which would be found in an individual with an unaltered hormonal state. All of the hormones are affected but the major changes are in the estrogens, progesterones and androgens. It should be emphasized that in the absence of local irritants clinically healthy gingiva will not show changes during these altered hormonal periods.

In pregnancy, the gingival changes are of two types, both of which may occur at the same time. The most common response is a generalized lesion with increased redness, swelling and bleeding of the gingival margin. This is generally more pronounced on the facial than on the palatal because the tongue cleanses the palatal area more effectively. The second type of response is a localized enlargement; an angiogranuloma of pregnancy ("pregnancy tumor"). These lesions result from severe local irritation and often occur with the more generalized type of response. Gingival changes in pregnancy usually appear during the second trimester. The microscopic changes in both types of lesion are similar but more clearly defined in the localized enlargement. The appearance is that of an angiogranulomatous reaction. There is increased capillary proliferation, dilation and engorgement of vessels, edema and degeneration in the connective tissue, proliferation and degeneration of epithelium and infiltration with leukocytes. The lesion tends to recur when removed unless the local irritants are also eliminated and prevented from returning. Estrogens and progesterones have varying effects on the tissues, among which are dilatation of peripheral blood vessels, increase in vascular permeability, increase in mitotic activity, and alterations in the ground substance with increased fluid retention. Changes similar to those occurring in pregnancy have been reported in women taking oral contraceptives and in some women during the menstrual cycle, particularly at times of ovulation when progesterones are highest. An exaggerated response to local irritants occurs in the gingiva of some children at time of puberty as a result of hormonal changes. It is found in both sexes but is more common in females. The histologic features are similar to those seen in gingivitis occurring in pregnancy.

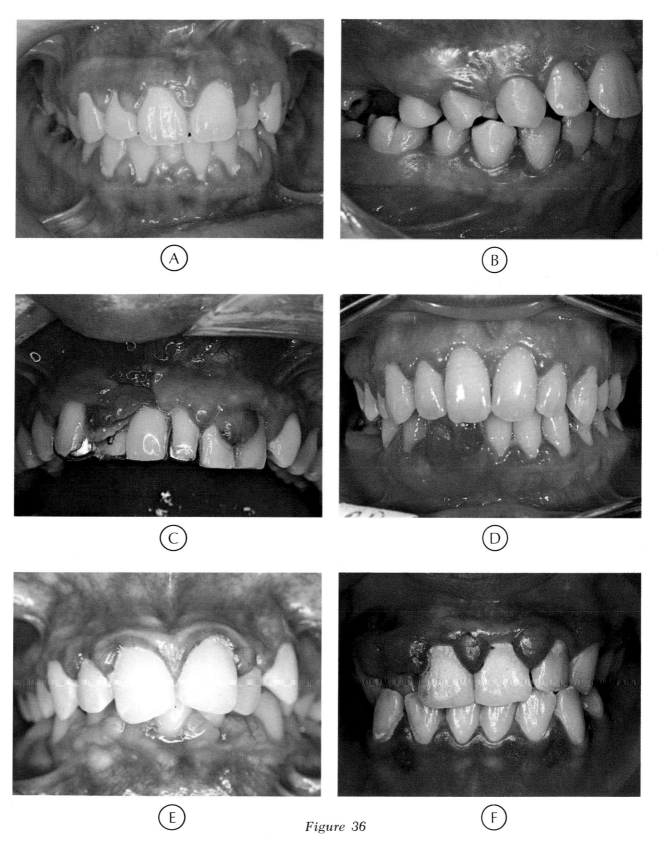

Figure 36

A-D. Gingival enlargement associated with pregnancy. In A and B, the enlargement is generalized and relatively uniform in size. In C and D, in addition to the generalized enlargement, there are discrete localized enlargements.

E and F. Gingival enlargement associated with puberty. In both pregnancy and puberty, the altered hormonal situation elicits an exaggerated response to local irritation.

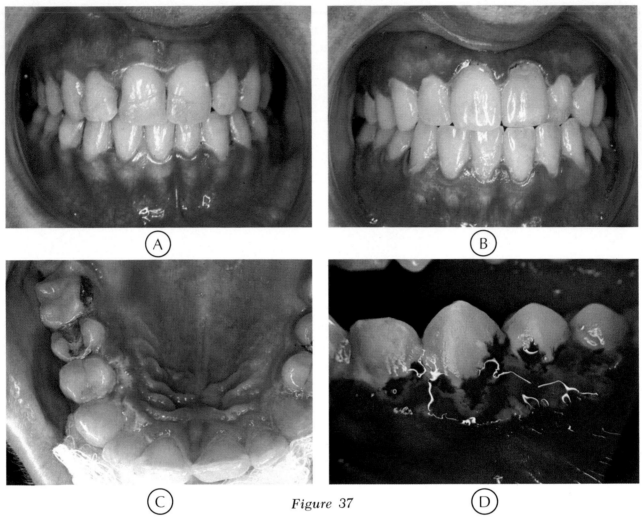

Figure 37

The patient illustrated in A has a slight to moderate case of ANUG with blunting of the papillae in some areas and necrosis with crater formation in others. B shows more advanced destruction with necrosis of the entire gingival margin of the maxillary central incisors. In C there is localized destruction of the palatal gingiva with extension onto the palate. In D there is a broad area of necrosis of the gingival epithelium leaving a gray pseudomembranous covering. Much spontaneous bleeding occurs from the exposed connective tissue.

ACUTE NECROTIZING ULCERATIVE GINGIVITIS

Acute necrotizing ulcerative gingivitis (ANUG), also called Vincent's infection and trench mouth, is the most common acute gingival disease. Its onset is sudden and often painful. Persistent mild cases are sometimes called subacute. The disease may be found generalized throughout the mouth but is frequently localized to one or a few teeth. Acute necrotizing ulcerative gingivitis is often recurrent and has a predilection for areas with deep periodontal pockets or malposed teeth such as lingually locked incisors. The clinical appearance of ANUG is characteristic. It presents as an erosion of the interdental papillae with a punched-out or crater-like depression in this area. The lesion is covered by a gray pseudo-membrane which forms from the necrotic tissue. Immediately surrounding these eroded areas the tissue is bright red. Spontaneous bleeding occurs from exposure of the connective tissue and subsequent rupture of the capillaries. The mouth has a foul odor and there may be increased salivation. The disease is usually superimposed upon an underlying chronic gingivitis but may occur in healthy mouths. The etiology has not been established. Smears of this condition yield increased numbers of *Bacillus fusiformis* and *Borrelia vincentii*, but these organisms are found in clinically healthy mouths. Acute necrotizing ulcerative gingivitis has not been demonstrated to be contagious.

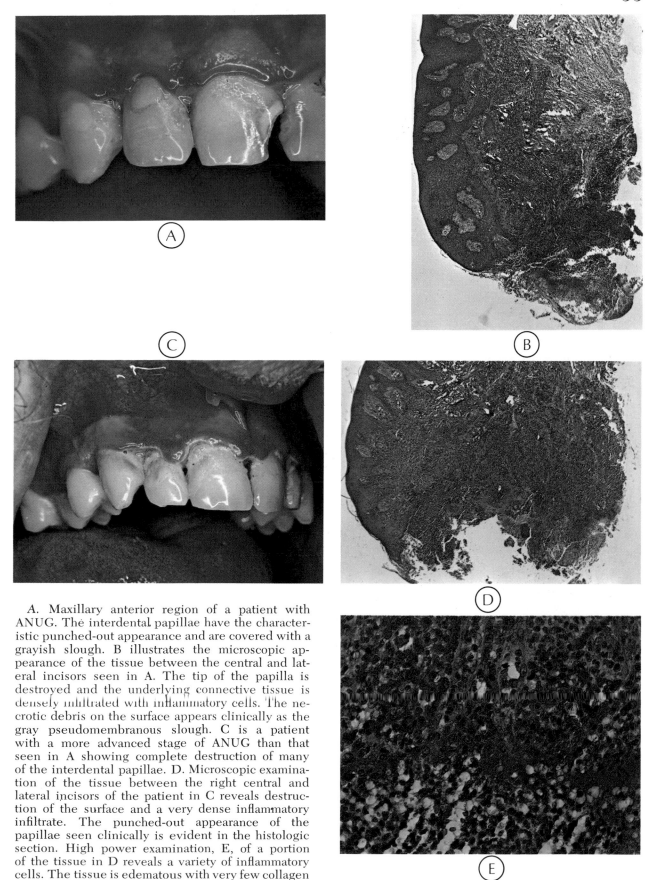

A. Maxillary anterior region of a patient with ANUG. The interdental papillae have the characteristic punched-out appearance and are covered with a grayish slough. B illustrates the microscopic appearance of the tissue between the central and lateral incisors seen in A. The tip of the papilla is destroyed and the underlying connective tissue is densely infiltrated with inflammatory cells. The necrotic debris on the surface appears clinically as the gray pseudomembranous slough. C is a patient with a more advanced stage of ANUG than that seen in A showing complete destruction of many of the interdental papillae. D. Microscopic examination of the tissue between the right central and lateral incisors of the patient in C reveals destruction of the surface and a very dense inflammatory infiltrate. The punched-out appearance of the papillae seen clinically is evident in the histologic section. High power examination, E, of a portion of the tissue in D reveals a variety of inflammatory cells. The tissue is edematous with very few collagen fibers remaining. There are numerous capillaries in this densely inflamed area.

Figure 38

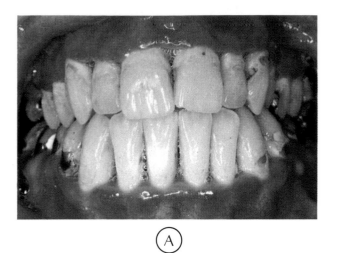

(A)

ACUTE NECROTIZING ULCERATIVE GINGIVITIS

Microscopically, ANUG appears as an acute inflammation of the marginal gingiva involving both epithelium and connective tissue. There is necrosis and ulceration of the epithelium with replacement by a fibrin network containing bacteria, leukocytes and necrotic epithelial cells. This debris forms the pseudomembrane. The connective tissue on the surface degenerates and in the surrounding area there is engorgement of capillaries and a dense infiltration with polymorphonuclear leukocytes. Since the microscopic appearance of ANUG is nonspecific and can be caused by burns, chemical or other injurious agents the diagnosis is based on the clinical findings.

The patient illustrated in A has ANUG which is most severe in the maxillary anterior region. In this area the interdental papillae have been destroyed, leaving a crater-like depression. In the mandible the blunted interdental papillae show the disease at an earlier stage. B illustrates the early stages of healing in tissue that is still densely inflamed. The epithelium is beginning to proliferate and grow underneath the necrotic surface in an attempt to protect the underlying connective tissue. C. Higher power examination of the proliferating epithelium seen in B shows a thin band of cells lining the inflamed connective tissue and walling off an area of necrosis. It will develop into mature stratified squamous epithelium. D is a high power area beneath the proliferat.. epithelium shown in C. There are numerous blood vessels and proliferating endothelial cells forming new capillaries. The area is heavily infiltrated with a variety of inflammatory cells.

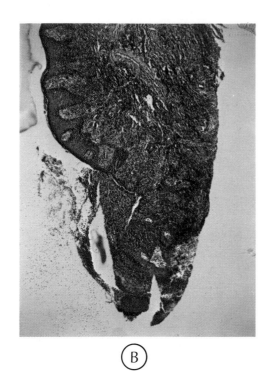

(B)

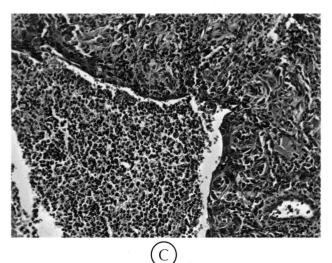

(C)

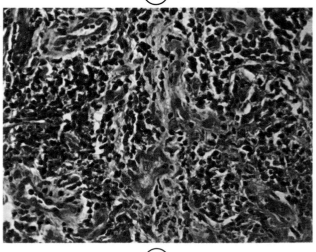

(D)

Figure 39

PERICORONITIS 57

PERICORONITIS

Third molars are often a direct cause of gingival and periodontal destruction in the retromolar area. Fully erupted third molars that are crowded or close to the ascending ramus may, because of these anatomic considerations, lack attached gingiva and a retromolar papilla. This lack of gingival tissue combined with the difficulty in cleansing in such an area leads to inflammation and destruction of the periodontal tissues. The partially or completely impacted third molar can be responsible for incomplete development or loss of fully developed supporting alveolar bone on the distal of the second molar. If the additional bone loss is combined with an already exisiting pocket, a more rapid destruction of the periodontal tissue occurs. In situations such as this, radiographs are extremely useful (Fig. 39A). When the third molar is partially erupted a space is present between the crown of the tooth and the overlying gingiva. This overlying gingiva forms a lid or covering called a pericoronal flap. This flap may also occur in fully erupted teeth when the tissue posterior to the third molar proliferates and covers a portion of the occlusal surface. An area such as this lends itself to impaction and retention of food debris and subsequent bacterial growth in the space between the tissue and the tooth. As a result, an infection termed pericoronitis may develop in the area. There is an influx of fluid and inflammatory cells; the tissues swell, appear redder and are painful. In the acute stage, the patient may not be able to bite properly because the swollen tissue extends above the occlusal line. The pain may radiate to the neck, throat and floor of the mouth. Associated lymph nodes may be enlarged and tender, the patient may have a fever and the infection may spread to other areas of the head and neck, most frequently the peritonsillar region. There may be an enlargement laterally which is usually confined by the buccinator attachment. This appears clinically as a swelling at the angle of the mandible. If the infection breaks through the anatomic barriers, it may spread via the fascial planes and anatomic spaces to more distant areas of the head and neck. The organisms most commonly associated with the development of infection are streptococci, staphylococci and Vincent's bacilli. If the infection is chronic, there may be virtually no discomfort to the patient. The undersurface of the flap is inflamed and there may be areas of ulceration in this region. Both acute and chronic stages may cause loss of periodontal tissues. The pericoronal flap area is often involved in acute necrotizing ulcerative gingivitis. Rarely, severe pericoronitis may lead to sequelae such as Ludwig's angina, cellulitis or peritonsillar abscess formation. *See illustrations on following pages.*

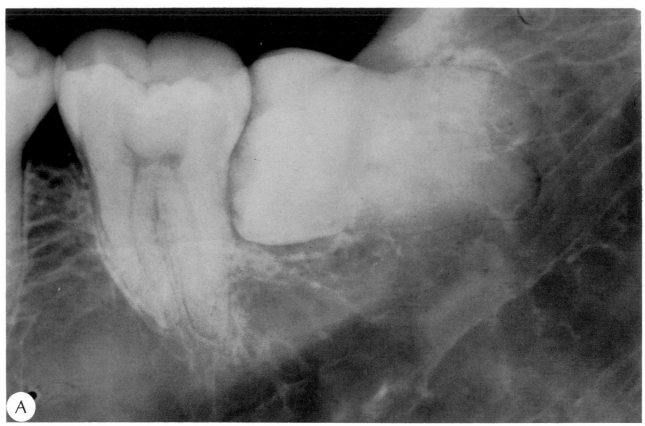

Figure 40

A. Radiograph of mandibular molar area showing horizontal impaction of third molar tooth. The crown of the tooth presses against the distal aspect of the second molar. There is no apparent root resorption but the alveolar bone distal to the second molar is much reduced in height.

B. Inflamed pericoronal flap (pericoronitis) covering disto-occlusal surface of mandibular third molar. Note swelling and fiery red color.

Figure 41.   See illustration on opposite page.

A. Microscopic appearance of tissue shown in radiograph in A. The empty area around the dentin of the crown represents the enamel which was dissolved during histologic preparation. Note pericoronal flap over impacted third molar.

B. Enlarged view of pericoronal flap shown in A. The tissue is dense and fibrotic and covered on the upper surface with stratified squamous epithelium.

C. High power of under (sulcular) surface of pericoronal flap. There is a dense infiltration of inflammatory cells in the tissue close to the tooth. The collagen fibers are being fragmented and destroyed. Numerous small engorged blood vessels are present.

D. Enlarged view of lower portion of impacted tooth seen in A showing dense connective tissue beneath the crown and reduced alveolar bone level in relation to the distal aspect of the second molar.

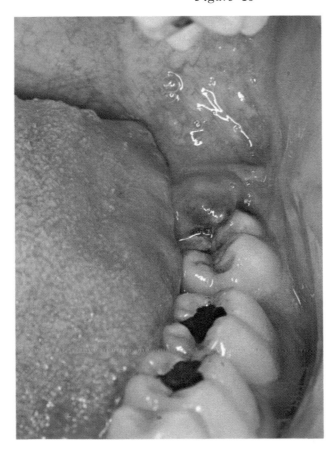

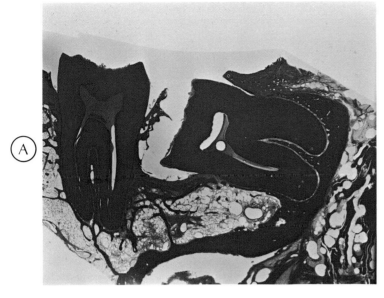

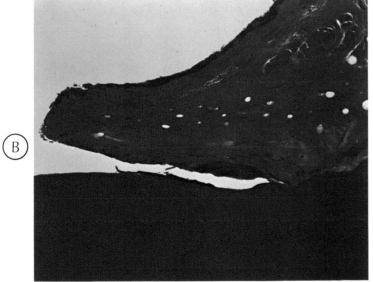

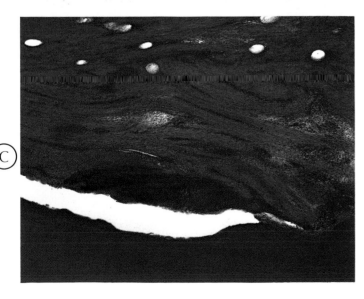

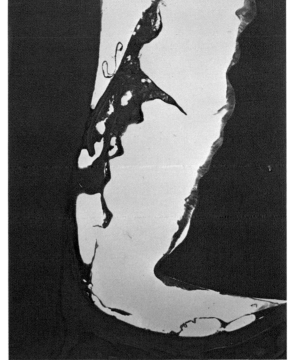

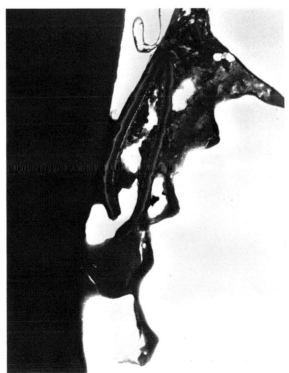

Figure 41

Legend continued.
   E. Higher power of debris between impacted third molar and distal root of second molar shown in D. Portions of the debris are adherent to a cuticular-like structure. The dentin is beginning to decay in this area.

ABSCESS

An abscess is a localized purulent inflammation which is associated with tissue destruction and liquefaction and is usually produced by pyogenic bacteria. There are three basic types of abscesses associated with the teeth and supporting tissues: (a) gingival abscess; (b) periodontal abscess; and (c) periapical abscess.

The gingival abscess is an uncommon lesion which is usually caused by a foreign body such as a toothbrush bristle or particle of hard food becoming embedded in the gingiva. It also occurs as a result of obstruction of drainage from a gingival cyst. Clinically, the lesion appears as a smooth, shiny, tense, red elevation in the marginal or papillary gingiva. If the lesion is fluctuant and pointing, the tip appears grayish-yellow from the pus; after bursting, a scab-like crust may form from the bloody discharge. During the interval prior to drainage, when the abscess is expanding most rapidly, the tooth may be sensitive to percussion. Since the gingival abscess does not involve bone, the radiographic findings would be negative.

The periodontal abscess (also called lateral or parietal abscess) arises apical to the gingival abscess in the underlying periodontal tissues and usually appears as a swelling on the lateral aspect of the tooth. Most often these lesions result from the obstruction of drainage from chronically inflamed tissues in a deep or tortuous periodontal pocket. Periodontal abscesses involve the periodontal ligament and frequently the alveolar bone as well. Clinically, they are similar in appearance to the gingival abscess. If the lesion is acute, the pain in the gingiva is throbbing and intense and may radiate to the surrounding areas. The tooth is mobile and is sensitive to percussion particularly in a lateral direction. When the lesion is chronic, a draining sinus is usually present. There is often a history of periodic acute flare-ups occurring when drainage from the sinus tract is temporarily blocked. This is followed by long periods of remission when the sinus is draining. During these periods of remission the patient may complain of a salty taste from the escaping fluid. At the opening of a draining sinus the tissue may proliferate to form an elevated nodule with a hole in the center which leads to a fistulous tract. More rarely, periodontal abscesses that are not involved with periodontal pockets may form. These usually present as swellings in the attached gingiva and result from root perforation during the course of endodontic therapy or from some other injury to the tooth and periodontal tissues.

The most common type of abscess is the periapical. It arises in the tissues at the apex of a tooth and is almost always due to the spread of infection from a diseased pulp. However, products from tissue break down or toxins from a sterile pulp necrosis can also be responsible for its formation. These abscesses frequently occur as acute flare-ups of periapical granulomas or cysts.

The systemic response to any abscess is quite variable. The ability of the host to localize the lesion is important and other factors such as age, general health and virulence of the organism play a role. The gingival abscess rarely has any systemic manifestations but the other types can cause complications such as fever, rapid pulse and general malaise.

The differential diagnosis between these lesions is often difficult, particularly when deciding between a periodontal and periapical abscess. One very useful test is tooth vitality. A tooth with a periapical abscess would be non-vital, those with a gingival or periodontal abscess would test vital. The periapical abscess is usually associated with deep caries or an extensive restoration. Entry into the pulp chamber and subsequent drainage of pus would indicate this type of lesion. Expression of pus from a periodontal pocket would be associated with a periodontal or gingival abscess. A tooth with a periapical lesion would generally be elevated in the socket and more sensitive to percussion in an axial direction. One with a periodontal lesion would not be elevated and be more sensitive to percussion in a horizontal direction. An exception to this would be a periodontal abscess in a furcation area, in which case the tooth would be quite sensitive to axial percussion.

Radiographs may not be helpful particularly in acute abscesses where the lesion has not had sufficient time to cause radiographically detectable bone loss. In long standing periodontal abscesses the most common radiographic finding is a widening of the periodontal ligament space or a radiolucent area in relation to the lateral surface of the root. If the lesion is interproximal and if it involves the bone it can be seen. If the abscess is buccal or lingual, it might be partially or totally obscured on the radiograph by the root of the tooth.

The differential diagnosis between these types of lesions depends on the case history and on careful interpretation of all available clinical and radiographic findings.

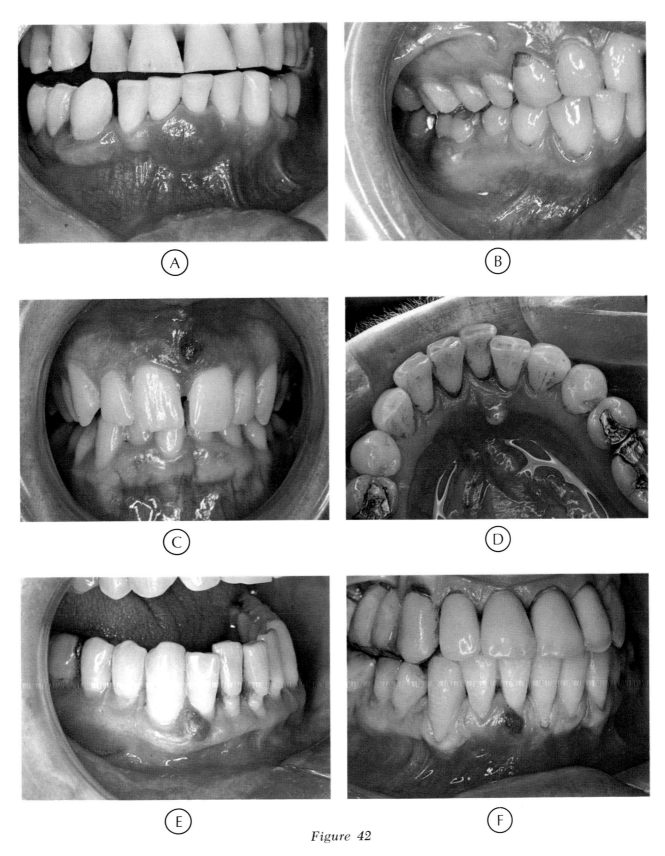

Figure 42

A to F. Periodontal abscesses in different locations and stages of development. In A and B, the abscess is acute and appears as a circumscribed swelling involving the mandibular incisors (A) and first molar (B). The gingival surface is smooth, red, shiny and tense. In C, E and F, the abscess is chronic and granulation tissue is present around the opening of the draining sinus. In D, the abscess is on the lingual surface, has pointed, and is about to drain.

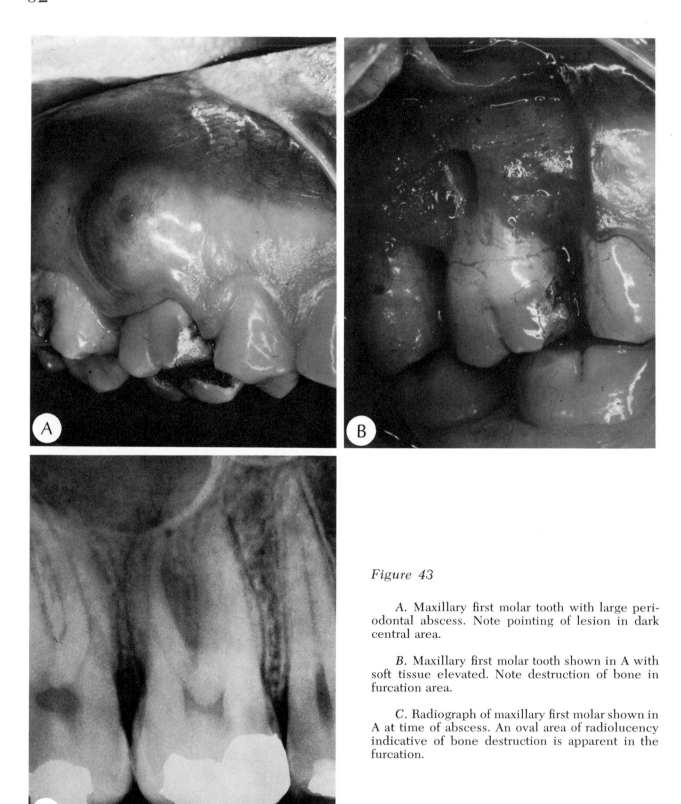

Figure 43

A. Maxillary first molar tooth with large periodontal abscess. Note pointing of lesion in dark central area.

B. Maxillary first molar tooth shown in A with soft tissue elevated. Note destruction of bone in furcation area.

C. Radiograph of maxillary first molar shown in A at time of abscess. An oval area of radiolucency indicative of bone destruction is apparent in the furcation.

Figure 44.   See illustrations on opposite page.

A. Radiograph of mandibular first molar and second premolar teeth. A large, oval, radiolucent area is apparent in the bifurcation of the first molar indicative of a possible periodontal abscess. There is pronounced reduction of bone height in the bifurcation. Note caries in both molar teeth.

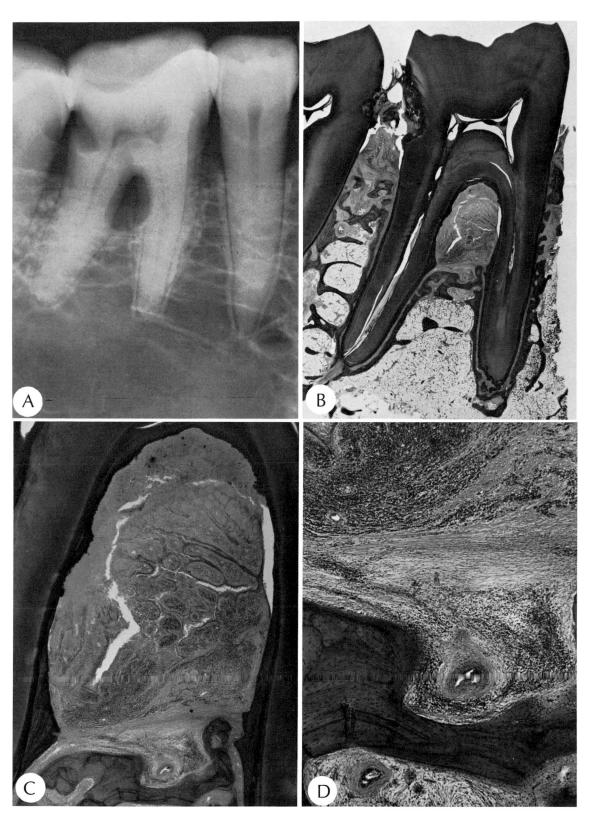

Figure 44

Legend continued.

B. First molar tooth shown in A. There is greater reduction of bone in the bifurcation than on the mesial or distal.

C. Higher power of bifurcation shown in B. A considerable amount of necrotic tissue is seen. The underlying connective tissue is heavily infiltrated with leukocytes and contains nests and cords of proliferating epithelium

D. High power of central portion of crest of bone in bifurcation shown in C. A dense inflammatory infiltrate engulfs the fragmented and degenerating collagen fibers. Two arterioles with thickened walls are noted in relation to the bone.

Desquamative Gingivitis

Chronic desquamative gingivitis is an uncommon gingival disease which in its severe form presents striking clinical features. It is seen more frequently in females than males, and occurs at any age after puberty, but most often after age 30. When this condition occurs in edentulous mouths, it is called desquamative stomatitis.

Chronic desquamative gingivitis is of indefinite duration with periods of remission and exacerbation, that may terminate spontaneously after months or years of involvement. It varies in appearance at different times and in different areas in the same patient. In advanced forms, the marginal and attached gingiva present an irregular distribution of bright red and gray areas, the surface is smooth and shiny and the normal resilience is replaced by a diffuse edema which pits on pressure (Fig. 45E). There are patches denuded of epithelium with an exposed bleeding connective tissue surface. The intervening areas are covered with gray friable epithelium which may be lifted from the surface or separated from it with a blast of air. In some cases, piled up epithelial strands formed in an effort at healing, cover most of the surface. Occasionally, vesicles develop (Fig. 45D) and rupture releasing a thin aqueous fluid. The pattern of gingival involvement changes as old denuded areas heal and new ones appear. In less severe forms chronic desquamative gingivitis presents diffuse erythema of the marginal and attached gingiva and diminished stippling (Fig. 45C). The labial gingiva is usually more severely involved than either the lingual or palatal gingiva. The gingiva on the palatal surface is often relatively uninvolved even in patients with severe changes labially (Figs. 45A and B). This difference appears to be related to local irritation. Tongue pressure and surface cleansing action of foods reduce the accumulation of irritating debris and inflammatory involvement on the lingual and palatal surfaces. The alveolar mucosa is usually abnormally shiny and hyperemic and there may be fissuring of the buccal mucosa at the line of occlusion.

Chronic desquamative gingivitis is often painless. However, some patients complain of a constant burning sensation, sensitivity to thermal changes, and cannot tolerate coarse foods and spices. Toothbrushing may cause painful denudation of the gingiva. Unwillingness to brush results in accumulation of irritating debris which aggravates the condition.

The prevalent opinion is that chronic desquamative gingivitis is a degenerative disease with secondary inflammatory changes. The inflammation is caused by local irritants such as plaque, starts in the gingival margin and extends to the attached gingiva. Another source of irritation is hot, spicy foods which are ordinarily well tolerated but become irritants because of the diminished protection provided by the atrophic epithelium.

The etiology of the noninflammatory degenerative changes is unknown. Insufficiency of gonadal hormones and nutritional deficiency have been suggested as etiologic factors. The degeneration occurs in the connective tissue and epithelium and may be systemically induced or secondary to locally caused inflammation. Chronic desquamative gingivitis sometimes occurs in patients with a history of hysterectomy at a young age or in post-menopausal patients, suggesting hormonal origin. However, most often the systemic history and laboratory studies provide no explanation for the oral changes.

The microscopic appearance varies in different patients and in different areas of the same patient. Atrophy and degeneration of epithelium and connective tissue, inflammation and attempts at repair occur to some degree in all cases but their distribution and severity vary. Subepithelial vesicle formation is a common but not universal finding.

It has not been established whether chronic desquamative gingivitis is a specific disease entity in itself or a clinical syndrome common to diseases such as bullous lichen planus, benign mucous membrane pemphigoid, or bullous erythema multiforme. Subepithelial vesicles are common in all of these diseases. The microscopic changes may represent a stage of these diseases or an unrelated gingival disorder.

There is a condition of the gingiva which resembles chronic desquamative gingivitis. It consists of diffuse erythema and desquamation of the gingiva caused by irritation from concentrated mouthwashes or hot foods. This is a simple response to local irritation, distinguishable from chronic desquamative gingivitis by the history, biopsy and the fact that discontinuing the offending agent results in uneventful recovery.

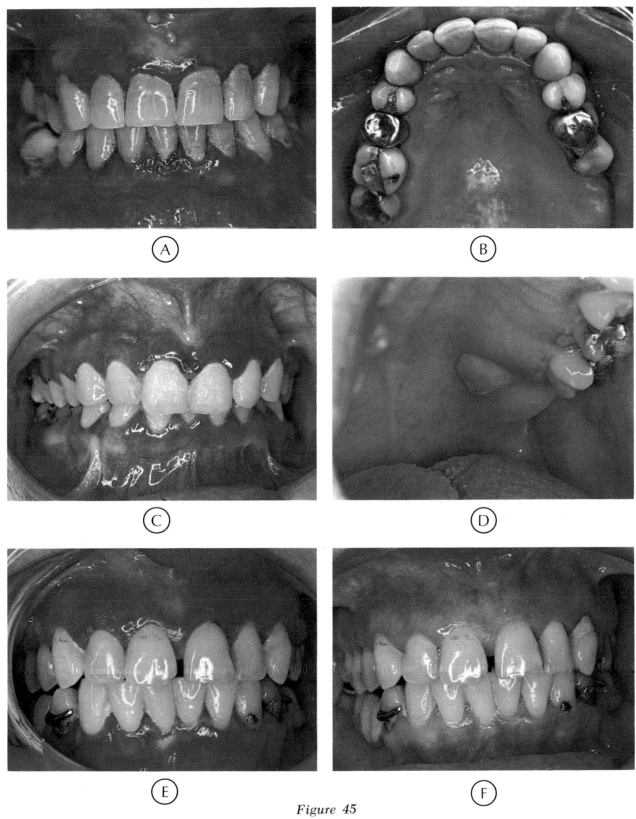

Figure 45

A. Severe chronic desquamative gingivitis involving the labial surface with diffuse erythema and desquamation of both marginal and attached gingiva.

B. Same patient as in A showing relatively uninvolved palatal surface.

C. Less severe chronic desquamative gingivitis.

D. Chronic desquamative gingivitis with bulla on palate.

E. Severe chronic desquamative gingivitis.

F. Same patient as E; 16 months after treatment.

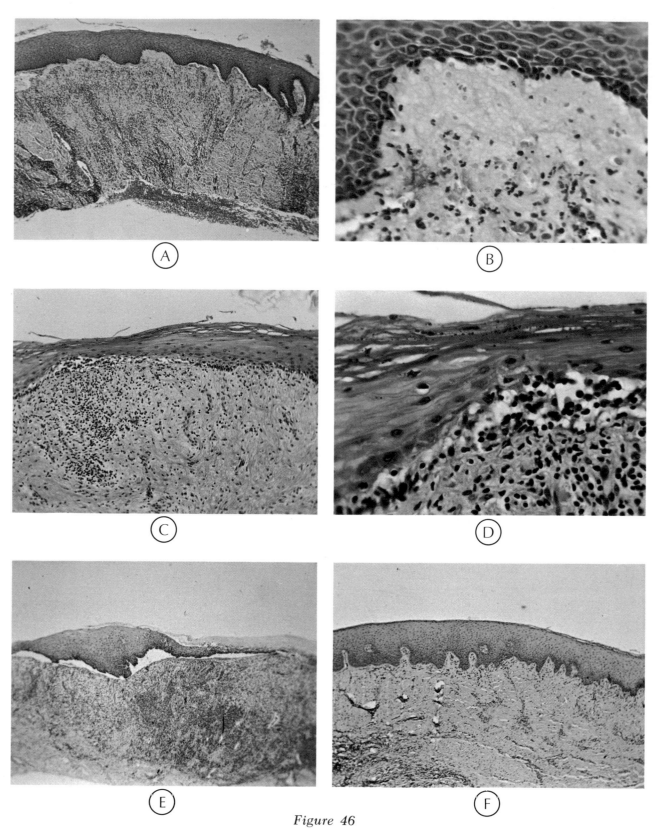

Figure 46

A–F. Histopathology of chronic desquamative gingivitis. A. Blunting of rete pegs. B. Detailed study of area in A showing replacement of connective tissue by inflammatory cells and fluid. C. Atrophy and degeneration of epithelium and inflamed connective tissue. D. Higher power of area in C showing microvesicle formation. E. Separation of epithelium from connective tissue and deeply penetrating inflammatory infiltrate. F. After treatment showing rete pegs beginning to repair and relatively normal histologic appearance; compare with E for before treatment.

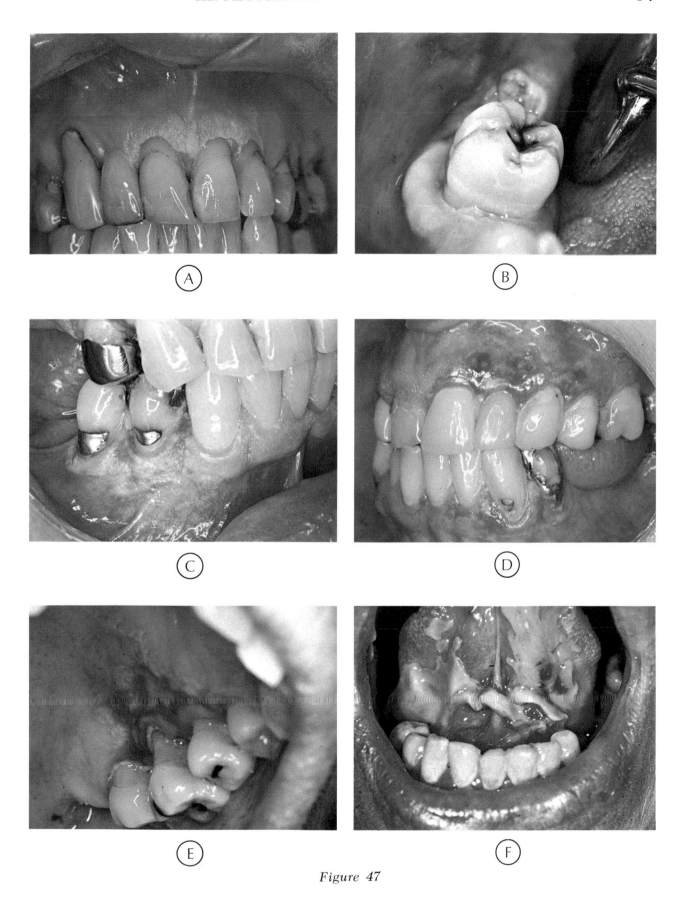

Figure 47

A-F. White and desquamating lesions. A. Hyperkeratosis above maxillary incisor teeth.
B. Thick, erosive leukoplakic type lesion around maxillary molar. C, D and E. Lichen planus.
Note erosions in D, more severe in E. F, Pemphigus vulgaris—note desquamation.

LEUKOPLAKIA—HYPERKERATOSIS

Leukoplakia is a general clinical term meaning "white patch." The lesions vary in appearance and texture from a fine white translucency to a heavy, thick, warty plaque. To be classified as leukoplakia, the lesion should be firmly attached to the underlying tissue and rubbing or scraping with an instrument should not remove it. It may occur anywhere in the mouth and is seen more frequently in males than females, usually in the middle-aged or elderly.

Hyperkeratosis or hyperparakeratosis are common histologic findings in leukoplakia. In hyperparakeratosis the granular layer is generally less well developed than in hyperkeratosis and in addition, the surface contains flattened, pyknotic, deeply staining nuclei. In both, there is hyperplasia of the epithelium and subsequent thickening (acanthosis) of the prickle cell layer. The epithelial ridges (rete pegs) proliferate and project more deeply into the underlying connective tissue. All layers of the epithelium, including the basal cells, remain intact. The connective tissue is diffusely infiltrated with inflammatory cells many of which are of the plasma cell type. As dyskeratosis may be one of the microscopic findings, biopsies should be done routinely for histologic evaluation.

The most frequent cause of hyperkeratosis or hyperparakeratosis is chronic mechanical irritation. This may result from a malposed or broken tooth or poorly fitting dental appliances. Smoking predisposes to leukoplakic lesions as does avitaminosis A. A condition known as white folded gingivostomatitis produces large leukoplakic type lesions. It is seen in children, usually has a familial history and persists throughout life.

Figure 48.   See illustrations on opposite page.

A. Marginal and attached gingiva showing epithelial hyperplasia, hyperparakeratosis and inflammatory cells in the underlying connective tissue.

B. Higher power of epithelium shown in A. Note pyknotic nuclei in the parakeratotic surface layer and moderately well developed granular layer with keratohyalin granules.

C. Hyperkeratotic lesion taken from buccal mucosa. There is a prominent granular layer just beneath the thickened keratin (right).

D. High power view of epithelium taken from same tissue block as C. Section stained with Barrnett-Seligman technique to show distribution of sulfhydryl groups. Note the dark staining sulfhydryl-rich "transitional" zone just above the granular layer.

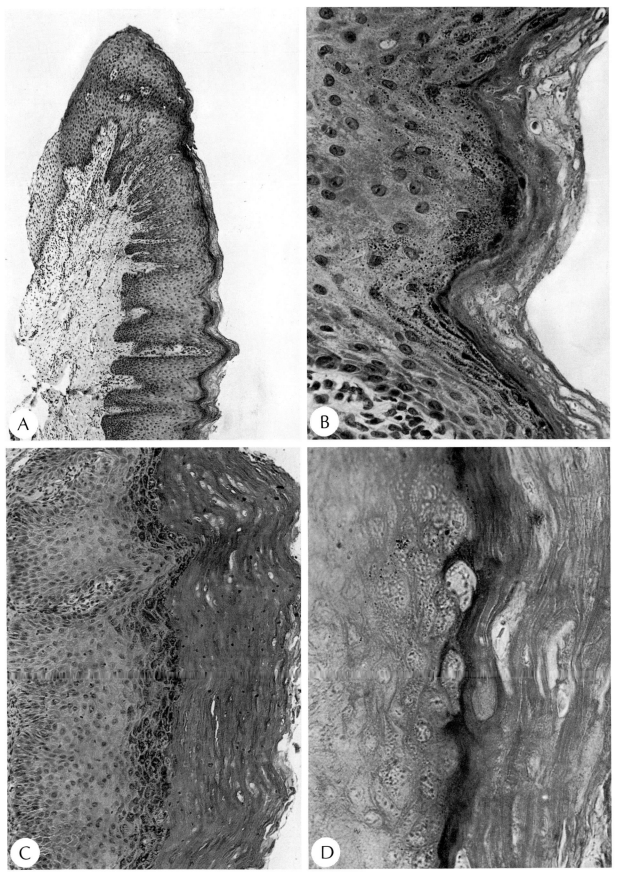

Figure 48

LICHEN PLANUS — PEMPHIGUS

Lichen planus is an inflammatory disease of skin and mucous membranes which clinically is characterized by small, shiny, punctate elevations along radiating lines or striae. The lesion frequently has a lace-like or woven appearance and is generally pearly-white to pinkish-violet in color. At times, the central area is dense and plaque-like and may be confused with leukoplakia. The periphery of lesions of this type is usually less dense and often shows the more characteristic appearance of lichen planus. Careful examination in this area may simplify making a differential diagnosis. Lichen planus is found in all areas of the oral cavity but is most common on the buccal mucosa. Itching may be a problem on the skin but does not occur in the mouth.

Microscopically, lichen planus is characterized by a dense band-like infiltration of leukocytes, mainly lymphocytes, in the connective tissue immediately subjacent to the epithelium. There is hydropic degeneration of the basal cells and frequently hyperplasia of the prickle cells (acanthosis). The granular and keratin layers may be thickened.

Several variations of lichen planus occur in the oral cavity. The most common is the non-erosive type which is generally asymptomatic. Other less common varieties are the erosive form in which there is atrophy, degeneration and in some areas complete absence of the epithelial covering. This type is generally painful. In some cases, the edema which is present in the connective tissue of all forms of lichen planus may be so extensive as to cause subepithelial bullae or vesicles. This variation is called bullous lichen planus. The etiology of lichen planus is not known but it may be associated with some form of emotional stress.

Pemphigus is a vesiculo-bullous skin disease which frequently has manifestations in the mouth. There are several varieties of pemphigus which include P. vulgaris, the most common type; P. vegetans, a variant of the vulgaris type; P. foliaceous and P. erythematosis. The latter two types rarely occur in the mouth. Pemphigus vulgaris occurs mainly in middle age. In more than 50 per cent of the patients, the earliest lesions occur in the oral cavity and later appear on the skin. All areas of the mouth may be affected. The microscopic appearance of this disease is characteristic. There is intra-epithelial vesicle formation and acantholysis (separation of individual and clumps of epithelial cells from one another.). The basal epithelial cells remain intact on the inflamed connective tissue which may contain a few eosinophils. The basal cell lamina junction remains intact because it contains the anchoring filaments of the connective tissue which are largely undisturbed. The epithelial cells above this layer depend upon the adhesive properties of the cell membranes and intercellular substances to hold them together. As a result of their degeneration, the epithelial cells separate from one another and an intra-epithelial vesicle develops. Indirect autoimmunofluorescence has demonstrated circulating autoantibodies and an autoimmune etiology has been postulated for this disease. However, at this time the etiology of pemphigus is unknown. Early diagnosis and treatment of this condition is imperative because if unrecognized and untreated, it may terminate fatally.

Figure 49.   See illustrations on opposite page.

A. Marginal and attached gingiva. There is a dense band-like infiltration of leukocytes immediately adjacent to the epithelium of the attached gingiva (left). The basal cells have degenerated and there is thickening of the keratin in this area. In the connective tissue below the sulcus (upper right) there is also an inflammatory lesion. However, in this area, the basal epithelial cells remain intact. The sulcular area shows the ordinary chronic inflammatory response while the attached gingiva has the characteristic lesion of lichen planus.

B. Higher power of the lesion of lichen planus shown in A. The basal epithelial cells (left) have degenerated or are undergoing degeneration. The dense band of leukocytes is mainly lymphocytes and some appear to have penetrated into the epithelium.

C. Pemphigus vulgaris. Most of the epithelium has separated from the underlying connective tissue by means of an intra-epithelial split. The basal epithelial layer remains intact and attached to the connective tissue. The underlying connective tissue is loose, edematous, and infiltrated with leukocytes. The epithelial cells are separating from one another indicative of acantholysis.

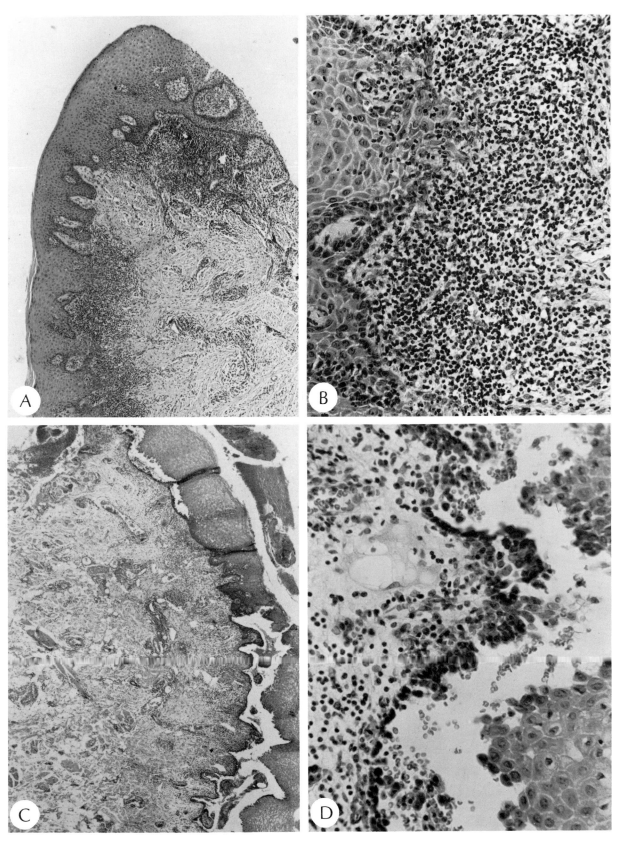

Figure 49

Legend continued.
   D. Higher power of lesion shown in C. The basal cell layer is still intact on the edematous connective tissue. Some of the epithelial cells (right) have separated from one another and are found in the vesicle space. Red blood cells and a variety of leukocytes are present.

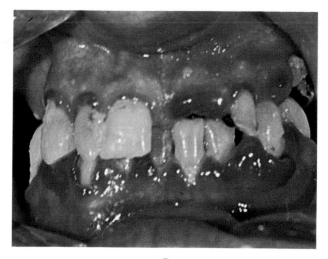

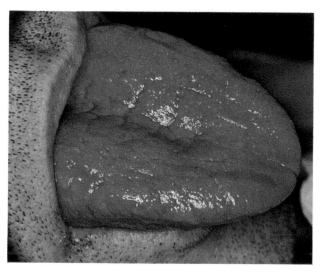

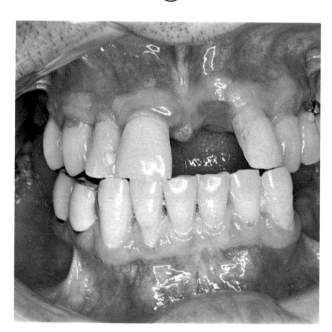

Figure 51

VITAMIN DEFICIENCY

Scurvy is a disease resulting from severe Vitamin C (ascorbic acid) deficiency. In the mouth, clinical signs of this condition include reddening and extreme friability of the gingiva, engorgement of blood vessels and loosening of the teeth. Vitamin C deficiency per se causes neither gingivitis nor periodontal pocket formation. Local irritants must be present for these to occur. However, it does exaggerate considerably the response to local irritation. In vitamin C deficiency there is arrest of collagen synthesis at the protocollagen stage and defective formation of the mucopolysaccharide ground substance. Capillary fragility is common due to the poor character of the connective tissue of the blood vessel walls. As a result of disturbances in connective tissue formation, healing is delayed. In contrast to the connective tissue changes, the epithelium appears relatively unimpaired.

In man, Riboflavin deficiency (Vitamin B₂) results in angular cheilosis, stomatitis and glossitis with depapillation of the filiform papillae. The tongue becomes smooth and red and may be painful. There are no apparent gingival changes. Similar oral lesions have been reported in animals with other members of the B complex group. As far as changes in the mouth are concerned, it is probably better to consider Vitamin B complex as an interrelated group rather than as individual components.

A. Chronic vitamin C deficiency. The marginal gingiva is enlarged, bluish-red and spongy. In some areas, the attached gingiva has the same appearance. A considerable amount of debris is present on the teeth.

B. Vitamin B deficiency of tongue and lips. The tongue is smooth, red, shiny and denuded of papillae. There is an angular cheilosis at the corner of the mouth.

C. Gingiva of the patient shown in B. The marginal and attached gingiva and alveolar mucosa show no characteristic lesions indicative of vitamin B deficiency.

ALLERGY — ABRASION — BURN

Hypersensitivity reactions may occur in the oral cavity either indirectly, as a result of systemic administration of an allergen, or directly, by local application of the agent to the tissues. The appearance of the lesion varies depending upon the severity of the response. The tissues become red, edematous and inflamed with varying degrees of vesiculation, sloughing and necrosis. Burning and itching sensations are common. Removal of the allergen allows healing to take place.

Overly vigorous use of the toothbrush may result in damage to the oral tissues particularly when it is combined with a highly abrasive dentifrice. In acute injury, the gingival epithelium is abraded resulting in a ragged and painful surface. Exposure of the underlying connective tissue will result in bleeding. A punctate appearance to the injury sometimes occurs especially when a new toothbrush with hard bristles is used. Adjacent freni are frequently bruised and irritated. Chronic toothbrush trauma may result in recession of the gingiva and exposure of the root surface with abrasion of the cementum and dentin. Teeth in buccal or facial version are more prone to this type of injury. Injudicious use of other oral cleansing devices such as toothpicks, dental floss and interdental stimulators may also cause trauma.

Burns from hot foods or chemicals may result in a non-specific type of acute gingival inflammation. The injury may be generalized or localized with involvement possible in any area of the mouth. The lesion is red, irregular in outline and covered in part with a grayish slough due to desquamation of the surface epithelium. Most frequently this type of injury occurs from extremely hot food or drink. Excessive use of undiluted mouth wash and the local application of aspirin to the gingiva in an effort to relieve toothache are common varieties of chemical burns. Questioning of the patient will generally reveal the offending agent. Healing is rapid and uneventful.

A. Acute allergic reaction to drug. Note redness and desquamation on palate and palatal gingiva.

B. Toothbrush trauma. Note redness and scuffing of gingiva and frenum in molar region.

C. Redness and ulceration of palate and palatal gingiva resulting from burn with hot food.

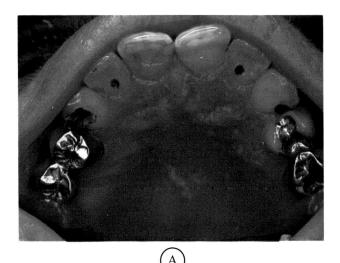

(A)

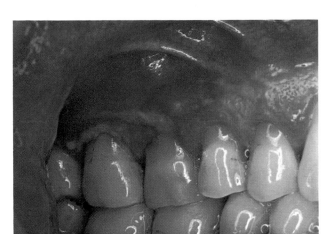

(B)

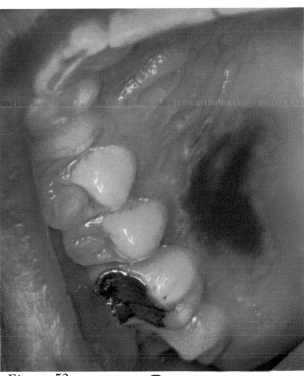

Figure 52   (C)

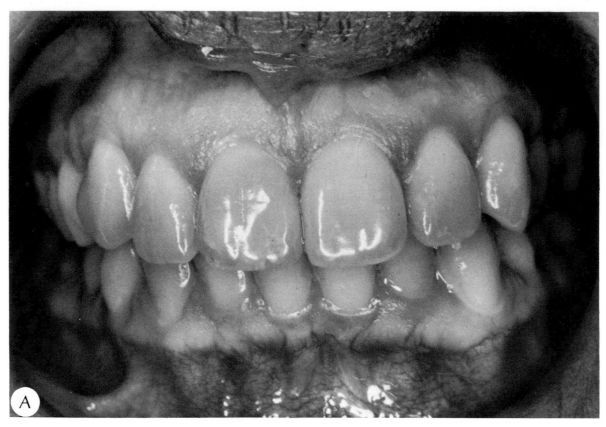

Figure 53

A. Patient showing slight marginal inflammation. There is some blunting and reduction in height of the interdental papillae and rolling of the gingival margin.

Illustration continued on opposite page.

Radiographic Appearance — Periodontitis

The radiograph is an important adjunct in the diagnosis of periodontal disease. It serves primarily for the detection of changes in calcified tissues. It does not, however, reveal very early bone loss nor does it show current cellular changes. An appreciable amount of bone destruction must have occurred histologically before it becomes apparent radiographically. The dense labial and lingual cortical plates often obscure the loss of inner cancellous bone thus allowing defects to occur without radiographic evidence of the destruction that has taken place. Examination of the bone with a probe is important as it provides a means for direct observation of the height and contour of the alveolus, particularly in the buccal and lingual areas, where the level of the bone may be obscured on the radiograph by dense tooth structure. The radiograph does locate areas of bone destruction but does not show whether a pocket is present in relation to these areas nor does it reveal the location of the epithelial attachment. Pockets must be determined by clinical examination with a probe.

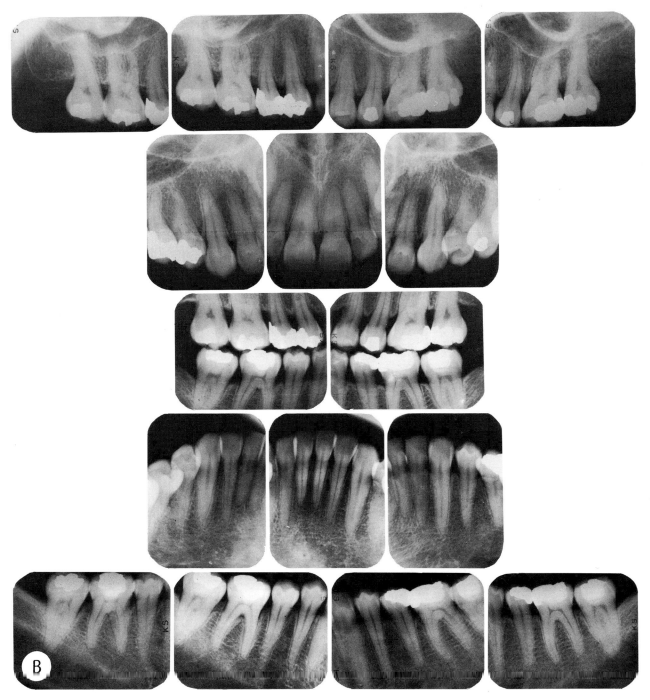

Figure 53

Legend continued.

B. Radiographs of patient shown in A. In the anterior region of both maxilla and mandible the alveolar bone appears slightly reduced in height. In the maxilla, there is reduction in bone height in the molar and premolar areas and widening of the periodontal ligament space mesial to the left second premolar. In the mandible, there is reduction in bone height and furcation involvement in the left first molar.

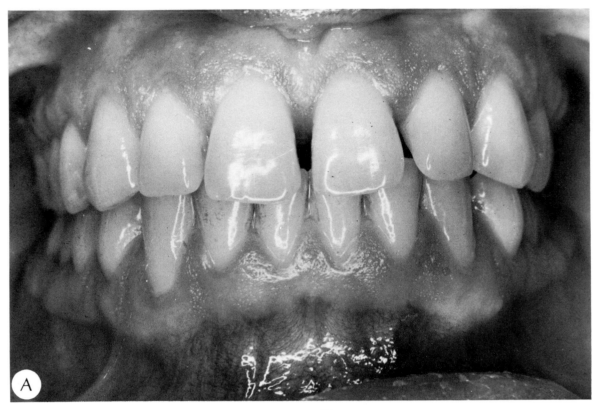

Figure 54

A. Patient showing slight to moderate marginal inflammation. Note the apparent recession in the maxillary anterior region. Stippling remains a prominent feature.

Illustration continued on opposite page.

RADIOGRAPHIC APPEARANCE—PERIODONTITIS

The earliest changes in periodontal disease are seen clinically rather than radiographically. The radiograph is an indirect means to determine bone loss. When properly used it reveals the current bone height. This must then be subtracted from the assumed normal bone height to determine the amount of bone loss. The age of the patient is an important consideration in determining the relative severity of the bone loss. If the same amount of destruction is present in a young individual and an old one, the relative tissue loss is greater in the former and the prognosis for the future course of the disease in the younger individual is less favorable.

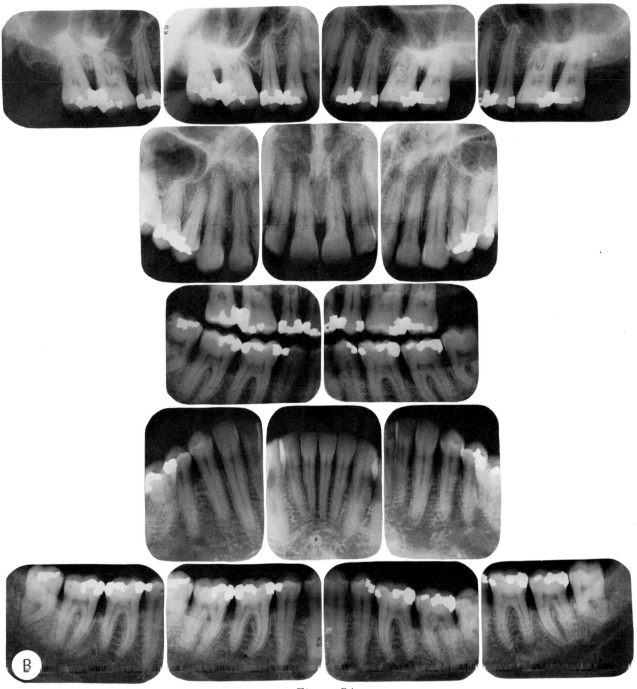

Figure 54

Legend continued.

B. Radiographs of patient shown in A. Bone loss is greatest in both maxillary molar regions with angular destruction and furcation involvement present in these areas. Bone defects are also noted distal to the left first premolar and mesial to the right lateral incisor. In the mandible, as in the maxilla, the greatest reduction in bone height is in the molar regions. Angular defects and furcation involvement are present in these areas. An angular defect is also noted mesial to the left second premolar. In general, however, alveolar bone loss is less pronounced in the mandible than in the maxilla.

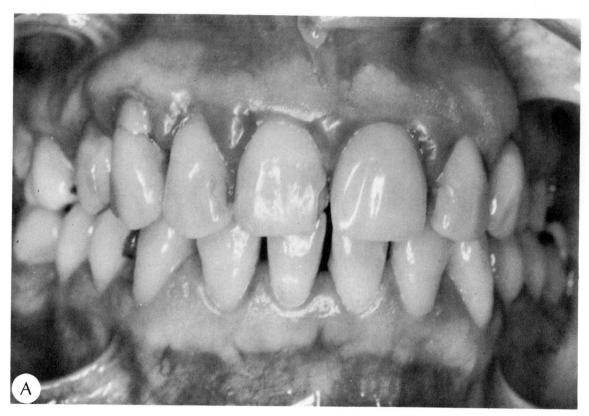

Figure 55

A. Patient showing moderate marginal inflammation. The gingiva in the maxilla, particularly in the interdental areas, is swollen and bulbous. The tissues are shiny and tense and there is loss of stippling. Note the relationship of the level of soft tissue to bone (B) particularly in the mandibular anterior region.

Illustration continued on opposite page.

RADIOGRAPHIC APPEARANCE—PERIODONTITIS

The radiograph reveals distribution of bone loss and this is helpful in determining the location of damaging local factors. The destructive process in periodontal disease may alter the contour of the interdental septum and create changes that affect the crestal lamina dura and the medullary spaces of the septal bone. The bone may be reduced in height in a plane which is perpendicular to the long axis of the tooth or in a direction which forms an angle or arc. In the former, the bone loss is termed horizontal and in the latter, angular or vertical. The earliest changes seen radiographically in periodontitis are a haziness and break in the continuity of the mesial or distal aspect of the crestal lamina dura. This results from the extension of inflammation into the crestal alveolar bone and subsequent loss of tissue. These changes are followed by a wedge-shaped widening of the interdental space and progressive reduction in height of the alveolar crest.

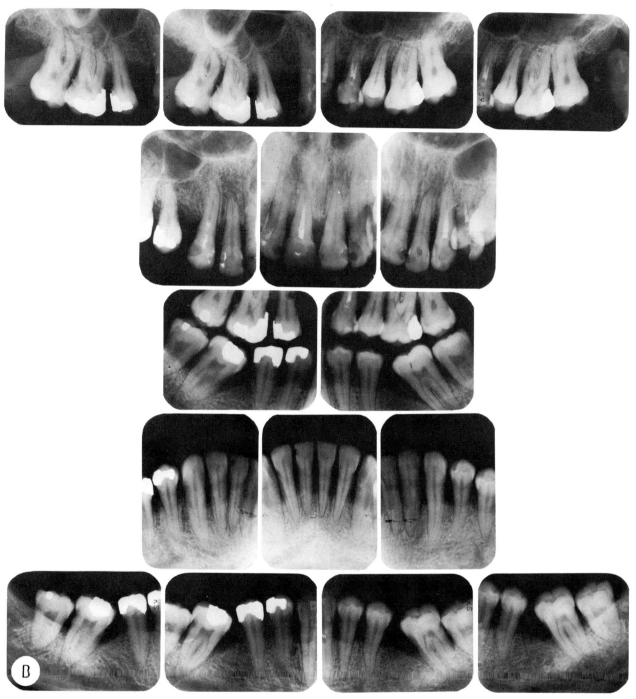

Figure 55

Legend continued.

B. Radiographs of patient shown in A. There is significantly greater bone loss than that seen in Figs. 53B and 54B. In the maxilla, the most severe bone destruction is seen bilaterally in the premolar and molar regions. All of the molar teeth have furcation involvement. In the mandible, the bone loss is greatest in the anterior and molar areas and least in the premolar region. Furcation involvement is present bilaterally in the molar teeth.

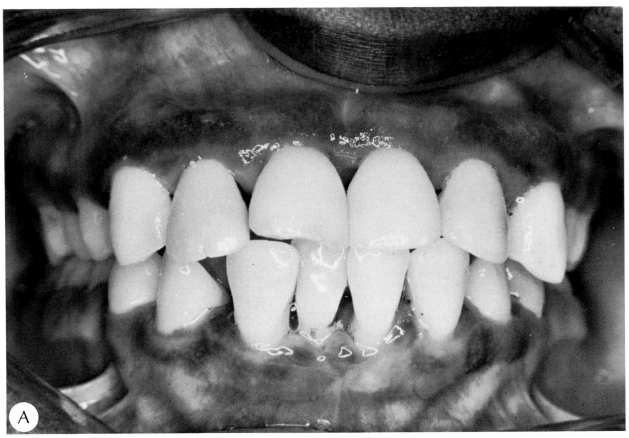

Figure 58

A. Fifteen-year-old female with periodontosis. The incisor teeth are migrating and the gingiva is inflamed. (Courtesy of Dr. Paul Baer.)

Illustration continued on opposite page.

PERIODONTOSIS

The radiographic features of periodontosis are fairly characteristic but not definitive. Bone loss is noted earliest in the incisor and first molar regions of both maxilla and mandible and it is in these areas that the destruction is most severe. Very often the bone loss is in an angular direction. Later there is generalized loss of bone throughout the mouth with the premolar area usually showing the least destruction. The bone trabeculae are often widely separated and poorly defined. Frequently, one or more of the first molar and incisor teeth are lost at an early age.

Histopathologically, the destruction of the periodontal tissues has been divided into three phases. The first is characterized by degeneration and desmolysis of the periodontal ligament fibers with cessation of cementum formation and resorption of alveolar bone. It is in this stage that the teeth begin to migrate. The second phase includes the rapid migration of the epithelial attachment along the cementum. Proliferation of epithelial remnants in the periodontal ligament may also occur and the first signs of inflammation are seen in this phase. Both first and second phases are of short duration and difficult, if not impossible, to separate clinically. During the third phase, the inflammation increases in severity and obscures the degenerative aspects. Large amounts of supporting tissue are lost rapidly. Periodontal pockets which were initiated during the second phase deepen and the teeth continue to migrate and become quite mobile. It is in this stage that the condition is usually recognized clinically. Many attempts have been made to establish a specific systemic or genetic background for this condition, but no specific cause and effect relationship has as yet been established.

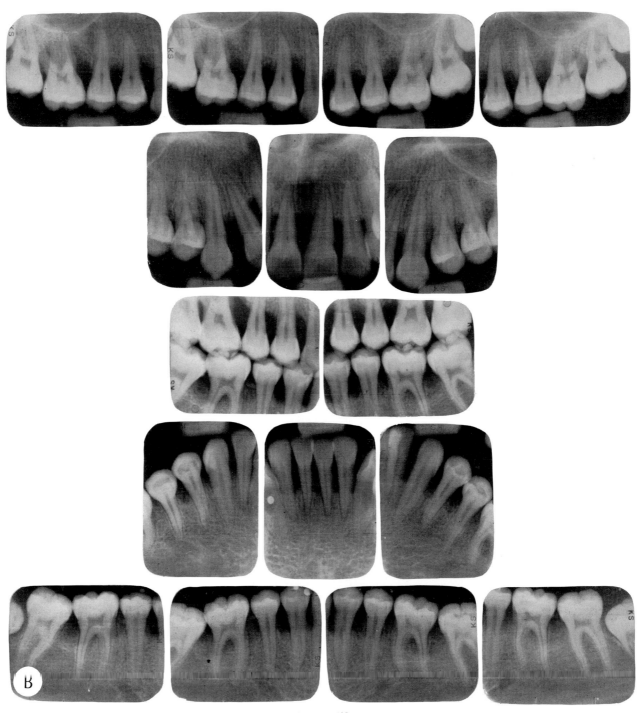

Figure 58

Legend continued.

B. Radiographs of patient with periodontosis shown in A. In the maxilla, there is severe generalized horizontal and angular bone loss most pronounced around the incisors and first molar teeth. In the mandible, there is generalized bone loss which is most severe in the incisor region. Angular bone destruction and furcation involvement are present about both first molars. Note generally thin roots and large bulbous crowns. (Courtesy of Dr. Paul Baer.)

PATHOLOGIC MIGRATION — DRIFTING — TOOTH MOBILITY

When periodontal disease causes an imbalance in the normal physiologic forces that maintain the proper relationship of the teeth to one another, a shift in their position occurs. This movement or shift in position is termed pathologic migration. In health, there are many factors which help maintain the teeth in a state of equilibrium. These factors include the periodontal tissues; the forces of occlusion; presence of a full complement of teeth; tooth morphology and cuspal inclination; pressure from the lips, cheeks and tongue; the physiologic tendency toward mesial migration; the nature and location of contact point relationships; approximal, incisal and occlusal attrition; and the axial inclinations of the teeth. Changes in any of these factors alter the complex interrelationship and may result in pathologic migration of one or more teeth.

Pathologic migration is a common finding in periodontal disease. It may be an early sign of the disease as in periodontosis or a later finding as in periodontitis. It is most frequently seen in the anterior region but is also found in the premolar and molar areas. Loss of the underlying tooth-supporting tissues and a force to initiate the movement are the two factors responsible for pathologic migration. A force which may have been acceptable to a tooth when the periodontal tissues were undamaged may be harmful to it when the supporting structures are weakened. The tooth now shifts its position in response to the force.

As the tooth migrates, the forces placed upon it are continuously changing. The migration will continue until a new equilibrium is established between the weakened periodontium and the occlusal forces. If the tooth is located in a position from which escape is not possible, the problem is compounded. The forces then aggravate and accelerate the loss of the periodontal tissues occurring as a result of the inflammatory disease. The pattern of bone loss may be altered resulting in crater formation and angular destruction and the inflammation from the gingiva may enter directly into the periodontal ligament.

Pathologic migration may occur on teeth that have no functional antagonist. Pressure from the muscles of the lips, tongue and cheeks may alter the position of a tooth. In addition, granulation tissue formed as a result of the inflammatory process in periodontitis also creates pressure which may cause migration. Extrusion may also be considered a type of pathologic migration. Lack of an opposing tooth combined with the continuous deposition of cementum permits the supra-eruption of the tooth. Loss of function owing to the absence of an occlusal antagonist results in atrophy and degeneration of the periodontal tissues.

Drifting should be differentiated from pathologic migration because in a strict sense they are not the same. The former occurs in teeth that are not involved with destruction of the periodontal tissues and in this regard differs from pathologic migration. Teeth often move or drift into positions that are harmful to the periodontium and as a result damage and tissue loss occur. When this takes place drifting becomes pathologic migration. Drifting frequently but not invariably occurs because of failure to replace a missing tooth or teeth. However, if, when a tooth is removed, the balance of forces on the remaining teeth has not altered sufficiently to require the establishment of a new equilibrium, their position remains unaltered. Teeth most frequently move in a mesial direction but it is not uncommon, especially for premolars, to drift distally. Along with mesio-distal movement, teeth may rotate and tilt or tip.

A certain degree of mobility is normal for all teeth. This movement is more pronounced horizontally than axially and greater for incisors than molars. Mobility is increased in individuals who brux or who have periodontal disease. The major reasons for pathologic mobility are loss of alveolar bone and other supporting periodontal tissues, injury from occlusion, and the presence of inflammation in the periodontal ligament. Mobility is temporarily increased after periodontal surgery, during pregnancy and in women who take hormonal contraceptives.

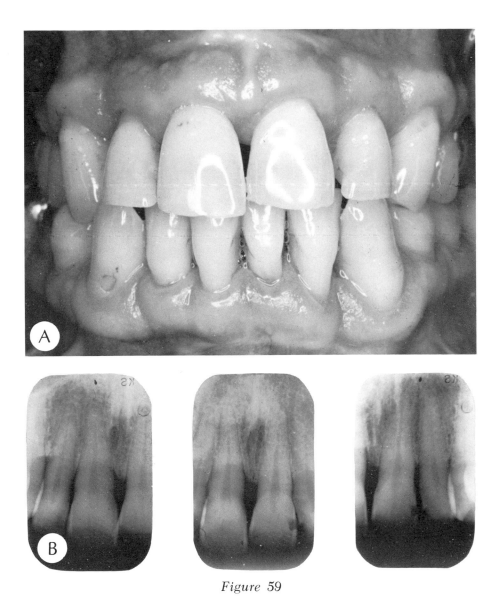

Figure 59

A. Patient with pathologic migration. The central incisor on the left has migrated anteriorly and extruded. The gingiva is bulbous and inflamed.

B. Radiographs of maxillary anterior region of patient seen in A. There is generalized horizontal bone loss with an angular bone defect on the mesial of the migrating central incisor. Angular or vertical bone defects are common around teeth with pathologic migration. They often result from the combined effects of inflammation and trauma from occlusion.

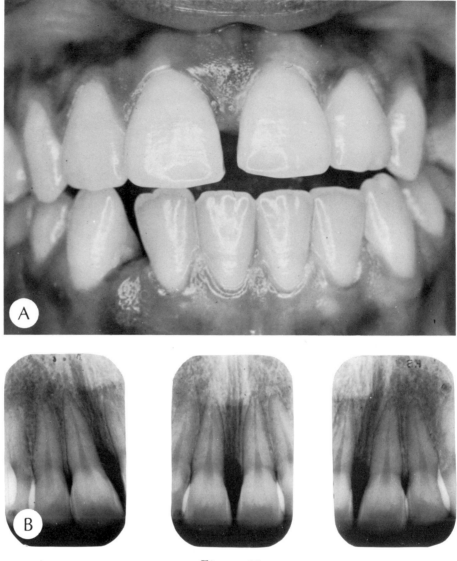

Figure 60

A. Patient with pathologic migration and extrusion of central incisor on the left. This is a more advanced stage than that seen in Fig. 59A. Note inflammation in the marginal gingiva.

B. Radiographs of maxillary anterior region of patient seen in A. There is an angular bone defect on the mesial of the migrating central incisor which is more pronounced than that seen in Fig. 59B. The adjacent teeth show only slight bone loss.

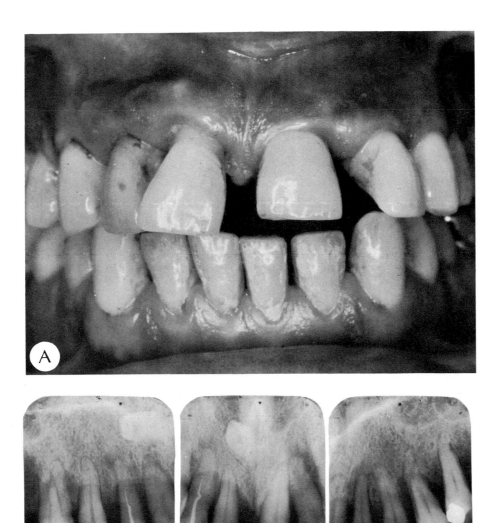

Figure 61

A. Patient with advanced pathologic migration and flaring of maxillary incisor teeth. The gingiva is inflamed and bulbous and the teeth are encrusted with heavy deposits of calculus.

B. Radiographs of anterior maxillary area of patient seen in A showing generalized severe angular and horizontal bone loss around all maxillary teeth. Note embedded supernumerary tooth above central and lateral incisors.

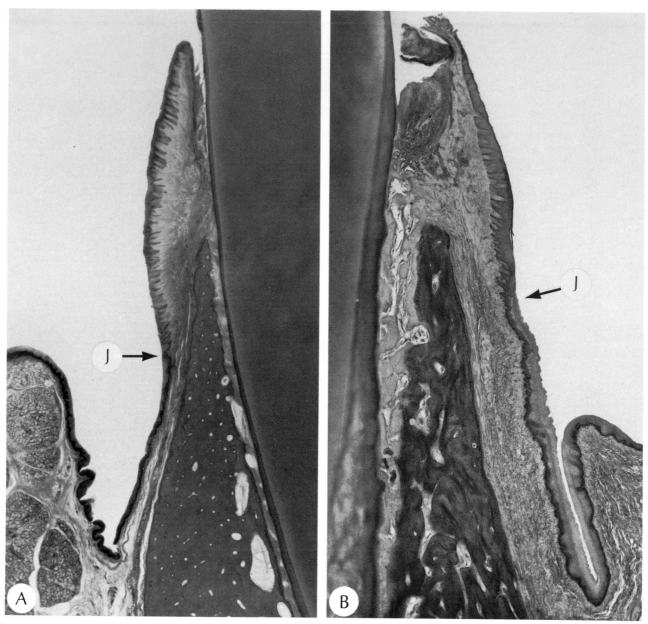

Figure 62

A. Lingual aspect of mandibular tooth showing inflamed marginal gingiva, attached gingiva, alveolar mucosa, vestibular sulcus and oral mucosa covering glands (left). The junction of the attached gingiva and alveolar mucosa (J) corresponds clinically to the mucogingival line. At this point, the epithelium loses its rete pegs and the connective tissue is areolar in type and does not contain the dense collagen fiber bundles present in the attached gingiva.

B. Buccal aspect of mandibular tooth showing similar histologic appearance to that seen in A. The glands noted in A are not present. A spicule of calculus is pressing into the pocket near the crest, causing inflammation and ulceration in the gingiva.

Illustration continued on opposite page.

Alveolar Mucosa — Hard Palate

The tissues of the alveolar mucosa differ from those of the gingiva and hard palate. The epithelium is non-keratinized stratified squamous and is thinner than that of the attached and marginal gingiva. The rete pegs are blunted or absent. The connective tissue is less dense and contains fewer collagen fibers. It is more loosely connected to the underlying periosteum and bone than the attached gingiva and may contain a few small, scattered, mucous glands. The surface of the alveolar mucosa is

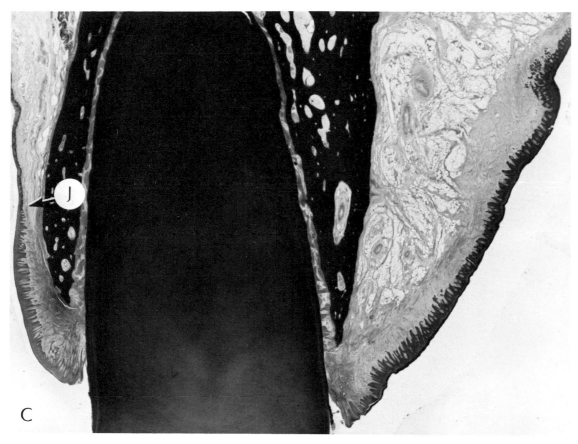

Figure 62

Legend continued.

   C. Bucco-palatal section of maxillary canine tooth. The junction (J) of attached gingiva and alveolar mucosa on the buccal is sharply demarcated. As in the mandible, the alveolar mucosa is thinner and does not contain the elongated rete pegs. There is no demarcation on the palate as the palatal gingiva blends imperceptibly into the palatal mucosa. In the anterior region, the submucosa of the palate contains much fatty tissue. In the posterior portion, there are numerous mucous glands.

smooth, shiny, softer in consistency and more red than the gingiva. It is quite vascular and this combined with the looseness of the connective tissue and thinner epithelium give the alveolar mucosa its characteristic red color. The region where the alveolar mucosa curves up to form the lining of the lips and cheeks is called the vestibular sulcus or fornix. The tissue covering these structures is attached to the underlying orbicularis oris and buccinator muscles respectively and contains small glands and fatty tissues. On the lingual surface, the alveolar mucosa reflects to become the lining of the floor of the mouth. The underlying tissues in this area contain numerous large and small salivary glands of both mucous, mixed mucous and serous types as well as fatty tissue.

   The mucosa of the hard palate unlike that of the alveolar mucosa is tightly bound down to the underlying periosteum and bone. It is the same color and texture as that of the gingiva. The epithelium is similar to that of the attached gingiva in that it is keratinized and contains elongated rete pegs. The incisive papilla is an elevated oval structure in the midline of the anterior portion of the palate just posterior to the maxillary incisor teeth. Extending posteriorly from this papilla, in the midline, is the median raphe. The rugae are ridges of dense connective tissue which extend laterally from the incisive papilla and the anterior portion of the median raphe. In man, they may be either symmetrical or asymmetrical. In the anterior portion of the palate, in the area between the median raphe and gingiva, the underlying submucosa contains much adipose tissue. In the posterior part of the palate, the adipose tissue is largely replaced by mucous glands. Bony growths or tori are frequently found in the palate particularly in the posterior region of the median raphe.

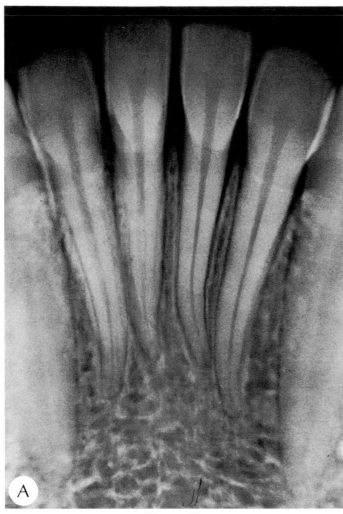

Figure 63

A. Radiograph of mandibular anterior region. There is slight, generalized horizontal reduction in bone height. The periodontal ligament spaces appear widened at the crest.

Figure 63B, C, D and E. See illustrations on opposite page.

B. Mesio-distal section of mandibular anterior teeth shown in A. There is a slight reduction in bone height with widening of the periodontal ligament in the coronal areas. Attachments for the mentalis muscle are seen between the canine and lateral incisor teeth.

C. Higher power of gingiva and crest of bone between left central and lateral incisors illustrated in B. The gingiva is inflamed and periodontal pockets are present on both lateral (left) and central (right) incisors. The gingival fibers are infiltrated with inflammatory cells and are degenerating. Calculus is attached to a cuticular-like structure which begins at the cemento-enamel junction and extends coronally.

VESTIBULE

The depth of the vestibule is an important clinical consideration in the examination of the mouth and is a factor to consider in the diagnosis and prognosis of periodontal disease. If the vestibule is shallow, there may be relatively little space for attached gingiva and as a result it may be quite narrow in width or even totally absent. Current opinion holds that the attached gingiva acts as a barrier to the deepening of a periodontal pocket and that an inadequate width or complete lack of this tissue will permit a more rapid apical extension of the disease.

In the mandibular anterior region, the point of origin of the mentalis muscle plays an important role in determining the depth of the vestibule. The mentalis is a short, heavy muscle that arises from the alveolar bone between the lateral incisor and canine teeth and extends to the chin where it inserts into the skin. It is located beneath the oral mucosa and as it reflects from the alveolus to the lips helps form the vestibule. If, by chance, the mentalis muscle is attached relatively high on the alveolar process its presence permits the development of only a relatively shallow vestibule.

In the posterior region of both maxilla and mandible, it is the buccinator muscle which is important in determining the depth of the vestibule. This muscle arises from the maxillary alveolar process in the molar region, the buccinator crest of the mandible, which is located on the alveolus in the area of the molar teeth, and finally from the pterygomandibular raphe of the buccopharyngeal fascia. The buccinator forms part of the cheek and is inserted primarily into the mucosa of the lips near the corner of the mouth. The vestibule in the molar region, particularly in the mandible, may be shallow because of a relatively occlusal origin of the buccinator muscle on the alveolus. In general, a shallow vestibule is more common in the mandible than the maxilla and more frequent in the posterior region than the anterior. A shallow vestibule is principally due to the positional relationship of the mentalis muscle anteriorly and the buccinator muscle posteriorly. When attempts are made to deepen the vestibule surgically, it is primarily these muscles that must be incised. Their cut surfaces must then be prevented from reuniting or the original shallow vestibular depth will recur.

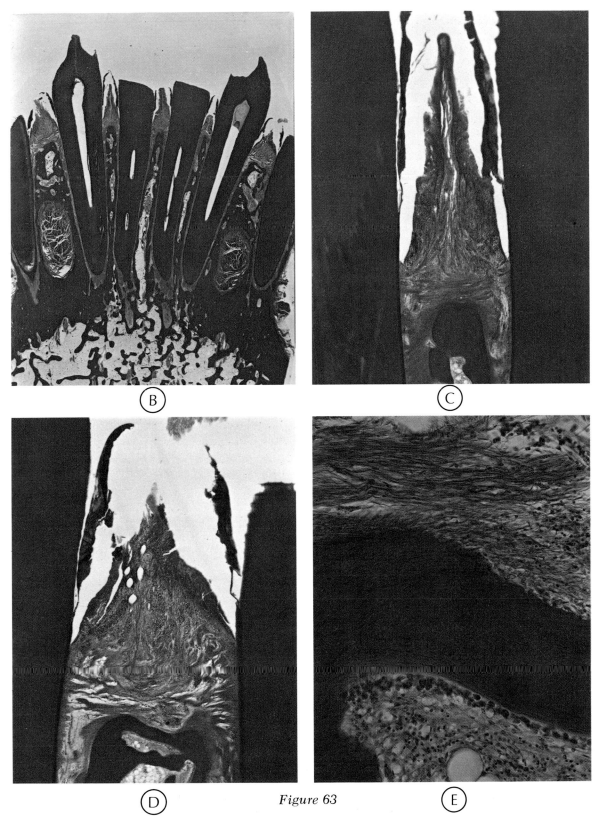

Figure 63

Legend continued.

D. Higher power of gingiva and crest of bone between right lateral (left) and canine (right) teeth illustrated in B. The gingiva is inflamed and the collagen fibers are degenerating. The crestal surface of the bone shows both formation and resorption. Bone is also being formed endosteally. Calculus is present and is attached in a manner similar to that seen in C.

E. High power of crestal bone illustrated in D. The collagen fibers are disintegrating and are infiltrated with leukocytes. The surface of the bone is being resorbed and has a ragged, scalloped appearance. The endosteal bone in the marrow space has a continuous layer of osteoblasts lining the newly deposited osteoid tissue.

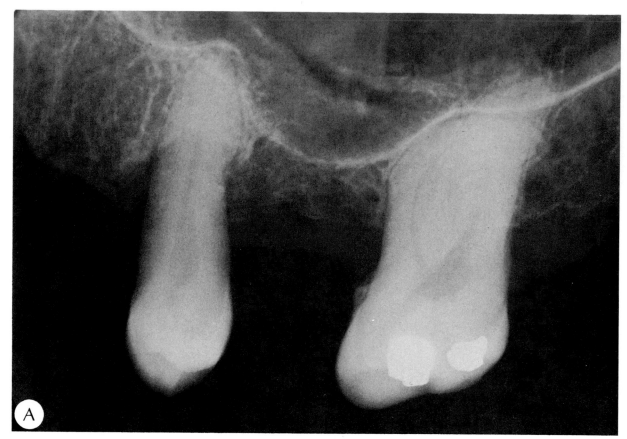

Figure 65

A. Radiograph of maxillary premolar and molar teeth. There is moderate to severe bone loss about both teeth with angular defects around the premolar. The heavy white line at the apex of the roots is the floor of the maxillary sinus.

RETROMOLAR AREA — MAXILLA

The maxillary tuberosity is covered by densely fibrous tissue called the maxillary tuberosity pad. This pad varies in thickness from a large prominence which may cover a portion of the occlusal surface of the tooth to a thin covering of tissue over the bone. The maxillary tuberosity or retromolar area becomes more prominent after eruption of the third molar. The bone surface is rough and contains a prominence called the alveolar tubercle which is formed by the two alveolar plates joining distal to the third molar. The tuberosity is bounded anteriorly by the distal of the last tooth and posteriorly by the hamular (retromolar) notch. This latter is a deep groove formed by the junction of the maxillary and palatine bones at the inferior border of the pterygoid process. Posterolaterally, the retromolar area is bordered by the attachment of the buccinator muscle and the superior attachment of the pterygomandibular raphe. Medially, it is limited by the soft palate and the tissues overlying the hard palate.

There are several anatomic considerations peculiar to this area which when combined with the difficulty of maintaining proper oral hygiene in this region may enhance the development of periodontal disease. Excessive fibrous tissue distal to the third molar makes cleansing in this location difficult and may allow for the development of a pathologic pocket. Exostoses may exist on both buccal and palatal alveolar surfaces and create ledges which favor the impaction of food and retention of debris. A shallow palatal vault may accentuate bony defects and complicate treatment. However, adequate cleansing by the patient will help reduce the incidence and severity of periodontal disease in this area.

Figure 65B, C, D and E. See illustrations on opposite page.

B. Mesio-distal section of maxillary molar and distal portion of premolar shown in A. The floor of the maxillary sinus is lined with bone which appears in the radiograph as a heavy white line. The bone distal to the molar is osteoporotic. An infrabony pocket is present on the distal of the premolar. There are thick dense pads of fibrotic tissue covering the bone.

C. Higher power of mesial pocket area of molar illustrated in B. The inflammatory response is confined mainly to the region beneath the hyperplastic epithelium lining the pocket. There is a large amount of calculus adherent to the cementum which in this area is acellular and thickened.

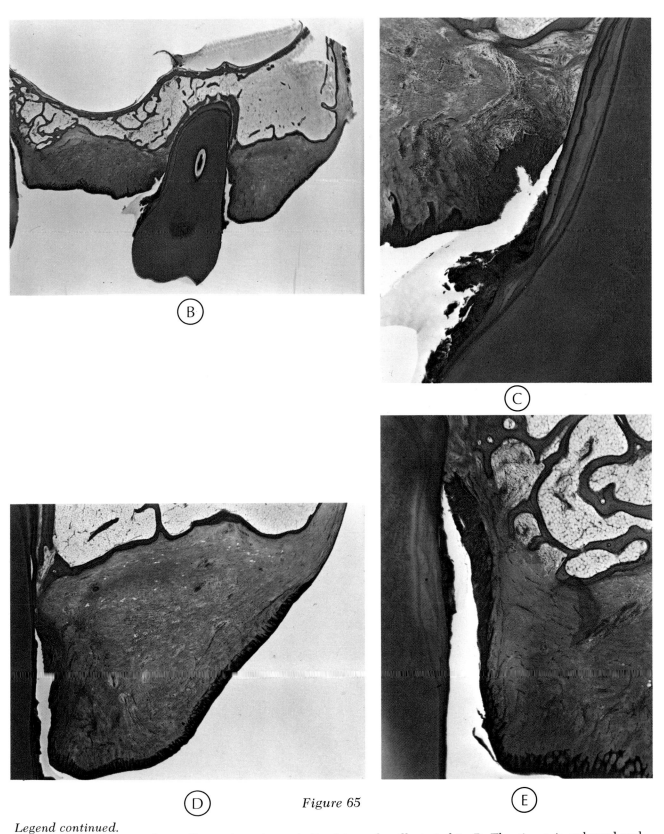

B

C

D

Figure 65

E

Legend continued.

   D. Higher power of maxillary tuberosity pad distal to molar illustrated in B. The tissue is enlarged and densely collagenous. The epithelium lining the pocket is hyperplastic. The inflammatory response is limited to an area immediately subjacent to the epithelium with the major portion being in the apical region of the pocket. Calculus is adherent to the cementum both supra- and subgingivally.

   E. Higher power of infrabony pocket on the distal of the premolar illustrated in B. The epithelium lining the pocket is hyperplastic. The leukocytic infiltration is slight and limited to the apical pocket area where it is seen entering directly into the bone. The connective tissue is hyperplastic and densely collagenous. A small amount of calculus is adherent to the cementum subgingivally.

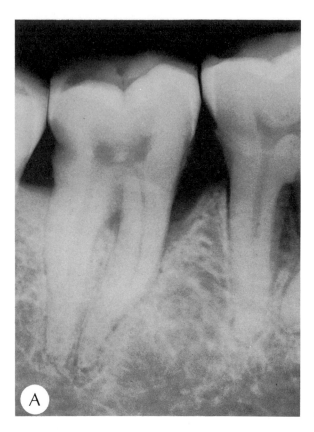

A. Radiograph of mandibular second molar showing angular bone loss on the mesial (right) and horizontal bone loss on the distal (left). Note bifurcation involvement and carious lesion on the distal.

Figure 66

CEMENTUM — CEMENTICLES

Cementum is a calcified tissue, similar to bone, that covers the roots of the teeth. Morphologically, there are two types of cementum, but chemically both are similar. The acellular (primary) type usually covers the coronal two-thirds of the root but may be found over the entire surface. The cellular (secondary) type is usually seen in the apical third of the root. An area of acellular cementum may be covered by the cellular type and these may alternate in almost any arrangement. Cementum is thickest on the apical third of the root and in the furcation region of multirooted teeth. Deposition of cementum, particularly in these areas, increases the length of the root and allows for continuous eruption of the tooth which, in turn, helps compensate for occlusal wear. The fibers of the periodontal ligament are embedded in the cementum and thereby form the main anchorage for the tooth in its socket.

Small fragments of calcified tissue, called cementicles, may be found free in the periodontal ligament or attached to the root surface. Frequently, they have a lamellated structure and contain cell-like inclusions which may be calcified epithelial rests. Cementicles are generally only a fraction of a millimeter in size but may coalesce to form larger structures. Increased thicknesses of cementum (hypercementosis), or spur-like projections (excementoses), may occur about a portion of one tooth or affect the entire dentition. This condition is usually found in teeth subject to increased function although it is occasionally seen on embedded or afunctional teeth. The additional cementum provides a larger area for attachment of periodontal ligament fibers and in this way gives greater anchorage.

Figure 66. See illustrations on opposite page.

B. Mesio-distal section of molar tooth shown in A. On the mesial, there is an angular bone defect with an infrabony pocket and on the distal, a suprabony pocket with horizontal bone loss. In the bifurcation, inflammation, loss of tissue and proliferation of epithelium are present. Note carious lesion in the distal of the crown.

C. Higher power of mid-portion of periodontal ligament distal to mesial root shown in B. There are numerous small irregularly shaped cementicles attached to the root surface and unattached (free) in the periodontal ligament. The surface of the adjacent bone is being resorbed.

D. Bone (left), periodontal ligament (center), and root surface (right) with two attached cementicles. The upper is lamellated and acellular; the lower, unlamellated with cellular inclusions.

E. Root surface with enamel matrix (arrow) between dentin (left) and hyperplastic cellular cementum (right). Above and below this area, acellular cementum covers the surface of the dentin. The adjacent periodontal ligament contains numerous small, irregularly shaped cementicles.

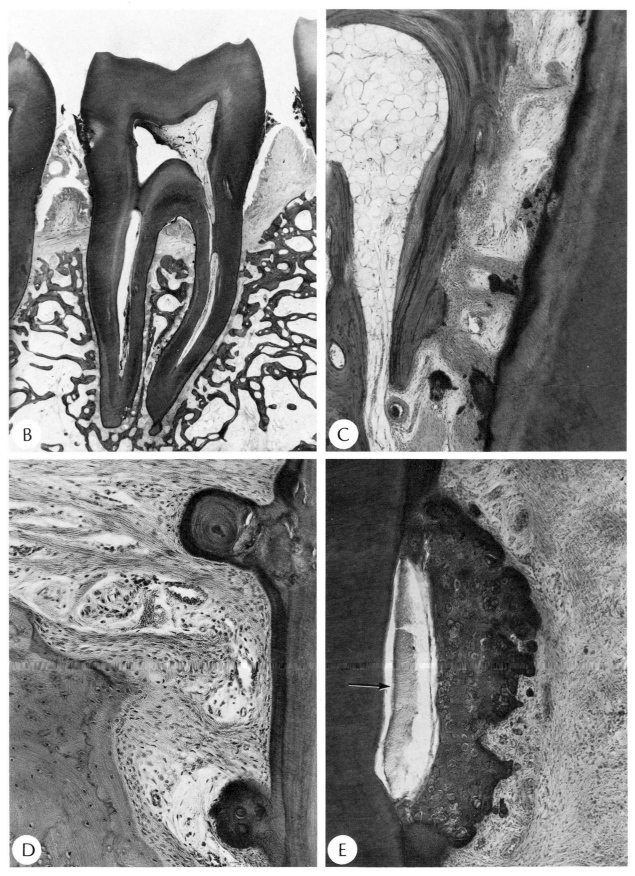

Figure 66

ROOT EXPOSURE – CARIES

Exposure of the root surface to oral fluids because of gingival recession or periodontal pocket formation results in degenerative changes in the cementum. Initially, the cementum has embedded in it Sharpey's fibers which are defined as that portion of the gingival or periodontal ligament fibers that are embedded in the cementum or bone. As the epithelial attachment migrates apically, the collagen fibers are detached and the root surface is covered with epithelial cells. During the detachment of the fibers, some of the cemental surface may be resorbed, because of decalcification and loss of matrix collagen. The epithelial cells continue their apical migration and as they do their coronal portion detaches from the root, leaving the cementum exposed to the saliva. Prior to their detachment these cells deposit the secondary dental cuticle on the tooth surface. The exposed cementum, which may be painful when brushed, or sensitive to hot and cold substances, may undergo additional degenerative and destructive changes. These changes include partial demineralization, softening, necrosis, resorption, greater roughness and increased permeability. Histologically, pathologic granules may develop. At times, exposed cementum may develop a highly mineralized zone on the surface. Inorganic minerals, such as calcium, which are present in the saliva, may precipitate on the tooth surface forming this hypermineralized region. This zone does not occur on all teeth nor cover all exposed areas of the same tooth. The hardness of cementum differs from tooth to tooth and even in different areas of the same tooth.

A bacterial plaque develops on the exposed surface and this may lead to caries of the root. Should this occur, the cementum becomes decalcified and the remaining matrix undergoes proteolysis. The cementum that is left becomes soft and necrotic and portions of it may fragment and chip away. The underlying dentin becomes involved in the carious process and saliva and bacteria penetrate the exposed dentinal tubules. One of the earliest destructive carious changes in the dentin is partial or complete demineralization followed closely by dissolution of the organic matrix from proteolytic enzymes. Just prior to this destructive process, the dentin becomes sclerosed. This is due to precipitation of minerals in the dentinal tubules in this region. As the carious process advances there is demineralization of the dentin further into the tooth with a still deeper penetration of bacteria in the dentinal tubules. Degenerative pulpal changes such as fibrosis and calcification may take place as a result of exposure of the root to the oral environment as well as from the carious process, and toothache may occur even though the crown of the tooth is intact. As in caries of the crown, sensitivity to sweets and thermal changes may be a problem.

There may be areas of osteoclastic resorption of cementum and dentin in teeth where the root is still covered with the periodontal tissues. These areas of resorption are generally repaired by deposition of new tissue and clinically present no problem. Occasionally, if the root becomes exposed prior to repair, these areas of resorption may be quite sensitive and require restorations. They can be differentiated from cemental caries by their well defined, sharp outlines and harder surface.

Abrasion and erosion which often occur after exposure of the root are similar in appearance. They present as smooth, hard, shiny, wedge or saucer-shaped depressions. Abrasion results from the mechanical wearing away of the tooth surface with some agent such as an abrasive dentifrice or denture clasp. The etiology of erosion is not known.

Figure 67. See illustrations on opposite page.

A. Radiograph of mandibular canine area. Arrows point to moderate caries on canine (left) and slight caries on first premolar (right) teeth. Note reduction in alveolar bone height.

B. Interdental area between canine (left) and first premolar (right). The gingival papilla is densely infiltrated with leukocytes and the upper portion is constricted by heavy calculus deposits adherent to both teeth. Note relationship of calculus to carious lesions.

C. High power of carious area of canine tooth shown in B. The cementum is destroyed and no longer apparent in this area except towards the bottom of the field where it is still present but undergoing necrosis. The dentin is decayed and the tubules enlarged. Filamentous bacteria are most prominent. Note their penetration directly into the tooth surface.

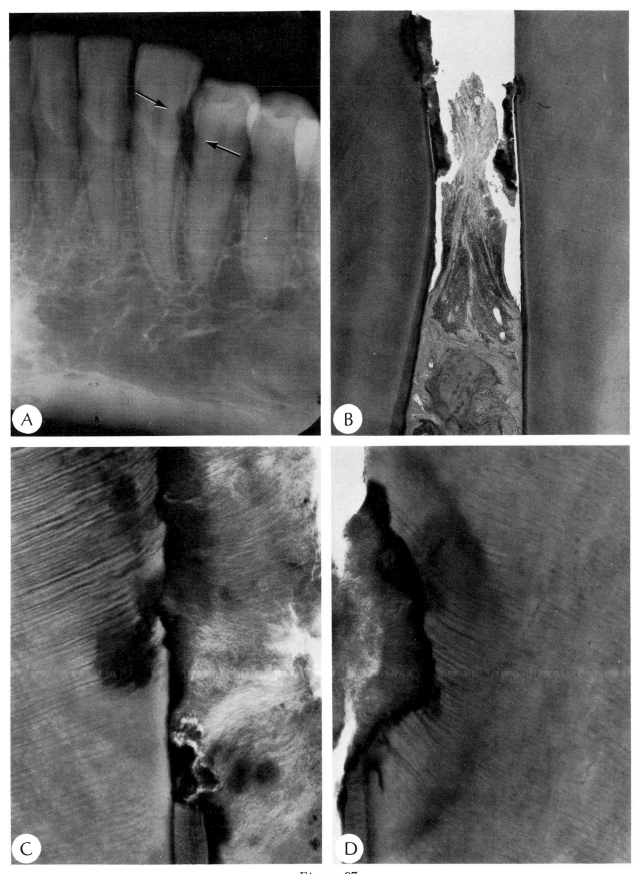

Figure 67

Legend continued.

D. High power of carious lesion in first premolar tooth shown in B. Both cementum and dentin have decayed, forming a saucer-shaped depression. The perimeter of future destruction is clearly defined by the dark semilunar outline surrounding the decayed area.

Periodontal Ligament Fibers

The collagen fibers of the periodontal ligament are subdivided into four major groups. The most coronal is the alveolar crest group which extends from the tooth to the crest of the alveolar bone. Immediately beneath these are the horizontal fibers that pass laterally from tooth to bone. The oblique fibers form the largest group. They extend from tooth to bone in a coronal direction and are located just below the horizontal group. The apical fibers pass from the apex of the tooth to the bone and compose the fourth group. Interspersed within the collagen fibers of the periodontal ligament are areas of a less dense areolar type connective tissue within which most of the cells, blood vessels and nerves supplying the ligament are found. The vascular supply to the periodontal ligament is derived from vessels coming from the alveolar bone, from branches of the apical vessels supplying the teeth, and from anastomoses with vessels from the gingiva. Small cords and nests of epithelial cells, which are remnants of Hertwig's epithelial root sheath and called epithelial rests of Malassez, are commonly found in the periodontal ligament. These cells may proliferate and form cysts, particularly when there is inflammation in the periodontal ligament. Small, round and irregularly shaped calcifications, derived from the cementum and called cementicles, may also be found in the ligament. The main function of the periodontal ligament is the attachment of the tooth to its socket. It also transmits the forces from the tooth to the alveolus and by this means aids in the remodelling of bone. The size and shape of the root, the number of fibers per unit area of tooth and bone, and the fact that the fibers are in a semi-fluid medium which acts as a hydrodynamic system are important factors in the transmission of these forces. The periodontal ligament forms a soft tissue covering surrounding the root and cushions the impact of tooth against bone. It also provides the cells that aid in its own maintenance as well as helping to supply the adjacent bone and cementum. In addition, it contains the blood vessels and nerves which furnish the necessary nutrients and sensation to the area.

There is a high turnover rate of protein in the periodontal ligament and probably a high turnover rate of collagen. The rate of collagen turnover along the bone is higher than that found in the midportion of the periodontal ligament, which in turn is higher than that found adjacent to the cementum. The highest turnover rate is located in the crestal and apical areas.

Figure 68.   See illustrations on opposite page.

A. Radiograph of mandibular second molar with mesial of third molar (left) and distal of first molar (right). There is moderate reduction in alveolar bone height with more advanced bone loss in the bifurcation of the second molar. Spicules of calculus can be seen radiographically on all teeth.

B. Mesio-distal section of molar teeth illustrated in A. Horizontal bone loss and suprabony pockets are present about all teeth. In the bifurcation of the second molar, there is inflammation with considerable reduction in bone height. Calculus is present in this area as well as around all teeth.

C. Higher power of interdental area between second and third molars shown in B. The gingiva is covered with calculus and is densely infiltrated with leukocytes. The transseptal fibers, despite the inflammation and bone loss, are well formed and form a dense band over the bone.

D. Higher power of interdental area between first and second molars shown in B. Despite the heavy inflammatory infiltrate, there are, in addition to the transseptal fibers, a few bands of gingival fibers extending from the tooth to the crest of the gingiva. Most of the gingival fibers have been destroyed but the transseptal fibers are a relatively constant finding in periodontitis and seem to re-form themselves more readily than do other gingival fibers.

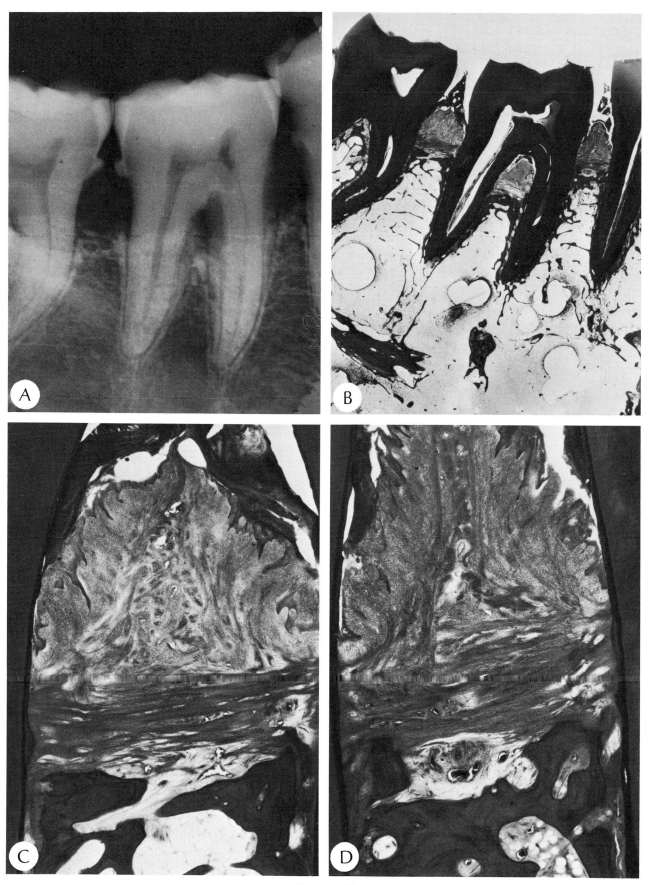

Figure 68

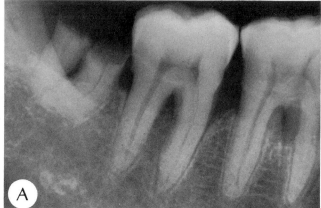

A

PERIODONTITIS – FIBROTIC GINGIVA

The evaluation of the gingiva is based on a thorough clinical examination which must include accurate probing of the sulcus or pocket. Frequently, the outer surface of the gingiva is firm, pink, stippled and fibrotic. This may be the result of the productive phase of an inflammatory process and not a condition of gingival health. Examination with a periodontal probe will demonstrate that there are pockets present and that these pockets will bleed readily. The inflammation may be confined to the inner portion of the pocket resulting in edema, leukocytic infiltration and degeneration of connective tissue in this area. The epithelium lining the pocket wall is, as a result of the inflammatory process, proliferating in some areas and degenerating in others. The tooth surface will have calculus adherent to it and there will be areas of rough and necrotic cementum. In contrast to the tissue adjacent to the pocket, the outer portion of the gingiva which is visible to the examiner may show a more fibrotic stage of the inflammatory process. Here the response is not the exudative phase of the inflammatory process with its edema and dense leukocytic infiltration, but the fibroplastic or proliferative phase with build-up of collagen fibers. There is only a slight infiltration of leukocytes and the epithelium is hyperplastic with elongation of the rete pegs. The superficial appearance is deceptive as it may give the impression of health when, in actuality, behind the wall of fibrotic gingiva, there is disease with destruction of the underlying tissue.

A. Radiograph of mandibular molar area. There is generalized reduction in bone height with furcation involvement in both first and second molars. Only the roots of the third molar remain.

B. Bucco-lingual section of jaw through distal root of mandibular first molar. There is inflammation in both buccal (right) and lingual (left) gingiva with reduction in bone height. Note calculus adherent to the tooth in relation to the gingival papillae. The mandibular artery and nerve are seen at N and the mylohyoid ridge at M.

Figure 69.   Illustrations continued on opposite page.

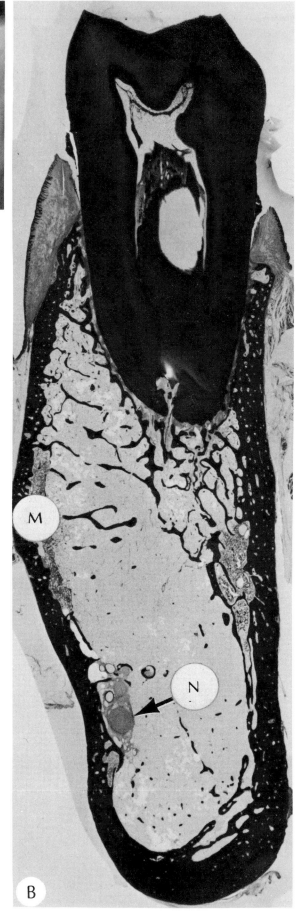

B

Figure 69

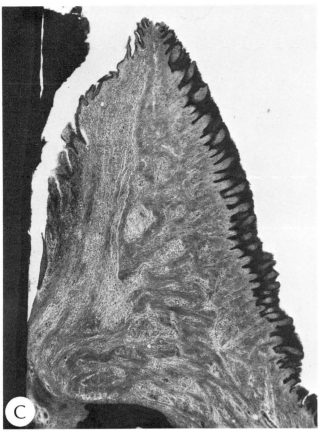

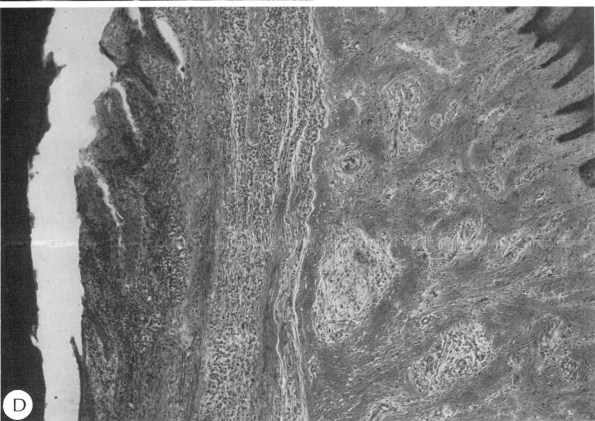

Legend continued.

C. Higher power of buccal gingiva and crest of bone illustrated in B. The connective tissue of the inner aspect of the gingiva is heavily inflamed and degenerating in contrast to the outer region which is densely fibrotic. Much of the epithelium lining the pocket is necrotic, resulting in ulceration while the epithelium lining the buccal surface appears relatively normal.

D. Higher power of gingiva illustrated in C showing sharp line of demarcation between the heavily inflamed inner aspect of the tissue and the densely fibrotic outer region.

Figure 69

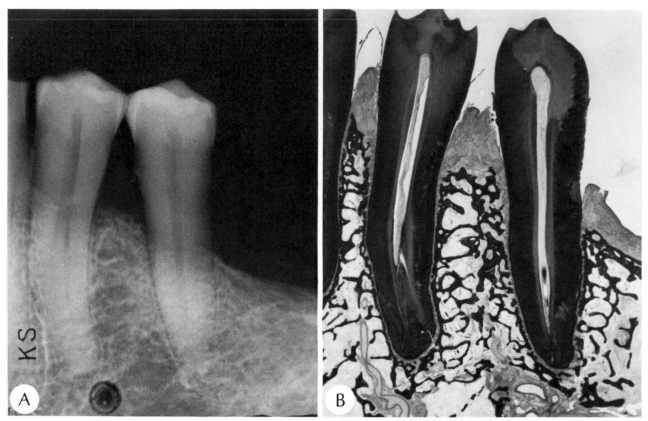

Figure 70

A. Radiograph of mandibular premolar area. There is reduction in bone height in the interdental region with apparent slight angulation of bone. In this case, the premolars are at different occlusal levels and the bone is parallel to a line drawn between the cemento-enamel junctions. As a result, the bone loss is considered horizontal, not angular.

B. Section of mandibular premolar area shown in A. There is angular bone loss between the canine (left) and first premolar teeth with a suprabony pocket on the distal of the canine and an infrabony pocket on the mesial of the first premolar. Between the first and second (right) premolars the reduction in bone height is horizontal. There are suprabony pockets present on the distal of the first premolar and on the mesial and distal of the second premolar.

PERIODONTAL POCKETS

A gingival sulcus that is pathologically deepened by disease is termed a pocket. It results from inflammation caused by local irritants. There are no systemic diseases which in the absence of local irritation will initiate pocket formation.

Pockets are classified according to their morphology and relationship to adjacent structures. Gingival (relative) pockets result from an increase in the bulk of the gingiva without destruction of the underlying periodontal tissues. They are found in gingival disease. Periodontal (absolute) pockets occur as a result of destruction of the periodontal tissues and migration of the epithelial attachment along with an increase in the bulk of the gingiva. They are subdivided into two types: (1) Suprabony (supracrestal) in which the base of the pocket is above the level of the alveolar bone and (2) Infrabony (subcrestal, intrabony, intra-alveolar) in which the base of the pocket is below the level of the alveolar bone. Both suprabony and infrabony pockets may be found in relation to the same tooth. Pockets are also classified according to the number of tooth surfaces they involve. Simple pockets involve one tooth surface and compound pockets, two. Complex (spiral) pockets follow a tortuous course around the tooth, involving two or more surfaces. The only accurate way to determine the presence and extent of a pocket is by careful probing. This should be done on all surfaces of the tooth in both a vertical and horizontal direction so as to avoid missing the compound and complex types.

A pocket is not constant in depth. It varies, shrinking and swelling, as fluids are lost or accumulate. The level of attachment of the base of the pocket on the tooth surface is of greater diagnostic significance than the depth of the pocket. Shallow pockets whose attachment is in the apical third are more of a problem and indicate greater severity of destruction than deep pockets whose attachment is in the coronal third.

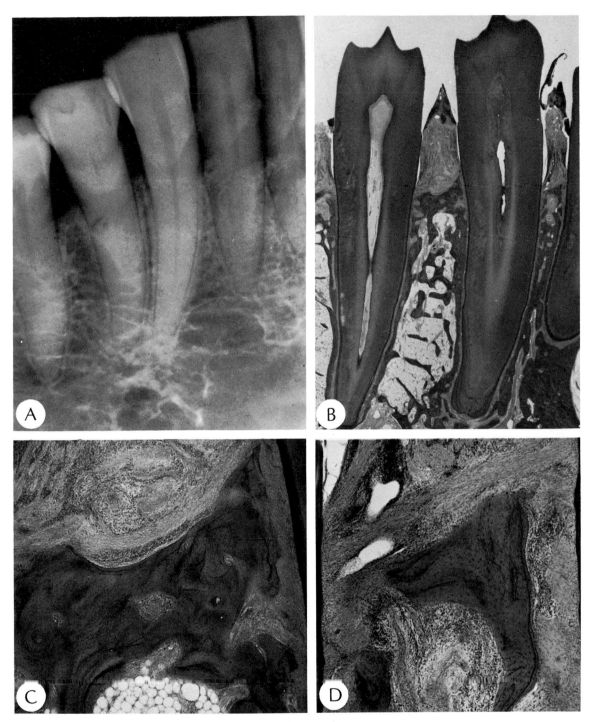

Figure 71

A. Radiograph of mandibular canine and premolar areas showing moderate horizontal bone loss.

B. Interdental areas between canine (right), first premolar (center) and second premolar (left) teeth shown in A. There is inflammation in the interdental papillae and reduction in the height of the alveolar bone.

C. Higher power of interdental crestal bone between first and second premolar teeth shown in B. Even though there is considerable inflammation present, new bone is being formed endosteally and on the crestal surface, particularly in the area adjacent to the periodontal ligament.

D. Higher power of interdental crestal bone between canine and first premolar teeth shown in B. Inflammatory cells are penetrating directly into the marrow space and are also seen in the periodontal ligament in relation to the early infrabony pocket (left).

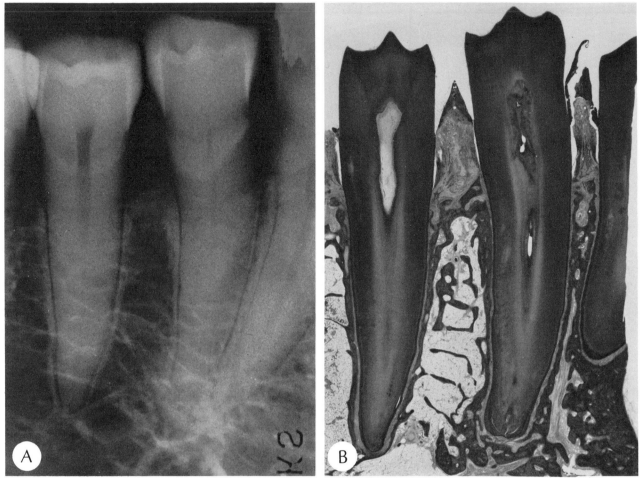

Figure 72

A. Radiograph of mandibular premolar area showing reduction in bone height and increased density of bone at the apices of the first premolar and canine teeth.

B. Mesio-distal section of premolar and canine teeth shown in A. There is generalized moderate reduction in bone height and considerable inflammation in the tissues. The bone in the area around the apices of the first premolar (center) and canine (right) teeth is more dense and relates closely to the radiographic appearance. Note suprabony pockets distal to the premolar and canine teeth and infrabony pockets mesial to both premolars.

See illustrations on opposite page.

C. Higher power of crest of interdental septum between canine and first premolar teeth shown in Fig. 72B. The inflammation from the gingiva enters directly into the crest of the alveolar bone.

D. High power of base of periodontal pocket and portion of crestal bone on mesial surface of first premolar shown in Fig. 72C. The inflammation is most severe in relation to the pocket wall. As it passes from the gingiva into the underlying bone it causes degeneration and fragmentation of the transseptal fibers.

PERIODONTITIS — SIMPLE AND COMPOUND

The extension of inflammation from the gingiva into the underlying alveolar bone and periodontal ligament is of major concern. It is at this point that gingivitis becomes periodontitis and the loss of alveolar bone and other supporting periodontal tissues begins. Since it is not possible to correlate the degree of inflammation in the gingiva with the exact time of extension of inflammation into the underlying periodontal tissues it is difficult to know precisely the point at which gingivitis first becomes periodontitis. To determine this, examination of the pocket with a probe to show that its base and epithelial attachment are on the root surface must be done. Periodontitis, the most common form of periodontal disease, is divided into two types: (1) Simple (marginal), resulting solely from inflammatory disease and (2) Compound, resulting from the combined effects of inflammation and trauma from occlusion. The radiograph is a useful tool for determining beginning bone loss and periodontal disease. However, since the earliest stages which are apparent histologically are not reflected in the radiograph it is possible to assume that if even a slight reduction in bone height is apparent on the radiograph, the actual histopathologic lesion has been present for a longer period of time and is more extensive.

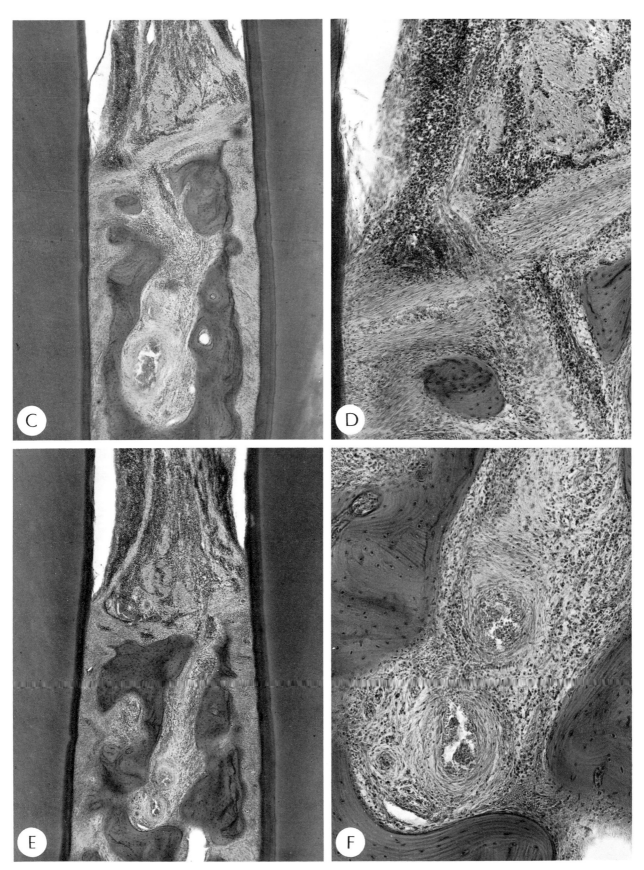

Figure 72

Legend continued.

E. Section taken from same block as tissue shown in C. The inflammation from the gingiva follows the vessels directly into the crest of the bone. Two arterioles are seen in the interdental bone.

F. High power arterioles seen in E. The walls of the vessels are thickened and the connective tissue surrounding them is infiltrated with leukocytes.

Pathway of Inflammation

The pathway of inflammation from the gingiva into the supporting periodontal structures is a critical factor in periodontal disease because it affects the patterns of bone destruction. Ordinarily, when inflammation spreads from the gingiva into the supporting periodontal tissues, the fluid and cellular exudate is found along the route of the vascular channels which seem to act as a path of least resistance. Animal experiments have shown that excessive occlusal pressure alters the alignment of the transseptal and alveolar crest fibers as well as the deeper fibers of the periodontal ligament. Excessive occlusal force also changes the pathway of the spreading inflammation so that it extends directly into the periodontal ligament, leading to angular resorption of the alveolar bone and infrabony pocket formation. Very severe excessive force produces necrosis of the periodontal ligament. The necrotic tissue acts as a barrier to the spread of inflammation until it is removed and the adjacent bone resorbed.

Findings in autopsied human jaws with periodontal disease corroborate the relationship between excessive occlusal force and the pathway of gingival inflammation demonstrated in experimental animals. The periodontal changes in humans are similar to those produced by excessive pressure artificially induced in animals. Interdentally, excessive occlusal pressure alters the alignment of the transseptal fibers as well as the deep periodontal fibers. Inflammation from the gingiva may then spread directly into the periodontal ligament. Infrabony pockets and angular or crater-like defects commonly occur around teeth with combined inflammatory and traumatic changes.

The pathways for the spread of inflammation from the gingiva to the underlying periodontal tissues may be described in the following manner:

Interproximally (Fig. 73E), the usual pathway is (1) directly into the crest of the bone and from there (2) into the periodontal ligament. Less frequently (3), when there is excessive occlusal force, it may go directly from the gingiva into the periodontal ligament.

Labio-lingually (Fig. 73F), the most common pathways for the inflammation are (1) along the periosteum, on the outer surface of the bone and then through the bone into the periodontal ligament or (2) directly into the crestal area of the bone and from there into the ligament. Less commonly, (3) the inflammation may go from the gingiva directly into the periodontal ligament. This latter pathway generally results when there is excessive occlusal force.

Inflammation in the periodontal ligament results in engorgement and dilation of the vessels, edema, leukocytic infiltration, degeneration of the connective tissue and resorption of bone.

Figure 73.   See illustrations on opposite page.

A. Radiograph of mandibular molar area. There is a slight reduction in bone height. The periodontal ligament space is widened along the mesial (left) of the second molar particularly in the crestal portion and the bone in this region is more dense. The glass cut indicates the plane of section shown in B.

B. Bucco-lingual view of mandibular second molar shown in A. The bone surrounding the tooth is composed of dense Haversian systems. There is a slight reduction in bone height on the lingual (left).

C. Higher power of lingual gingiva and bone shown in B. Much of the inflammation is confined to the marginal gingiva. However, there is some extension of inflammation into the underlying tissue.

D. Higher power of crest of bone and gingival fibers illustrated in C. Inflammatory cells are seen passing over the crest of the bone. They do not penetrate directly into the periodontal ligament. Note relatively well formed gingival fiber bundles.

E and F. Diagrams illustrating the pathways for the spread of inflammation from the gingiva into the underlying periodontal tissues. See above for description.

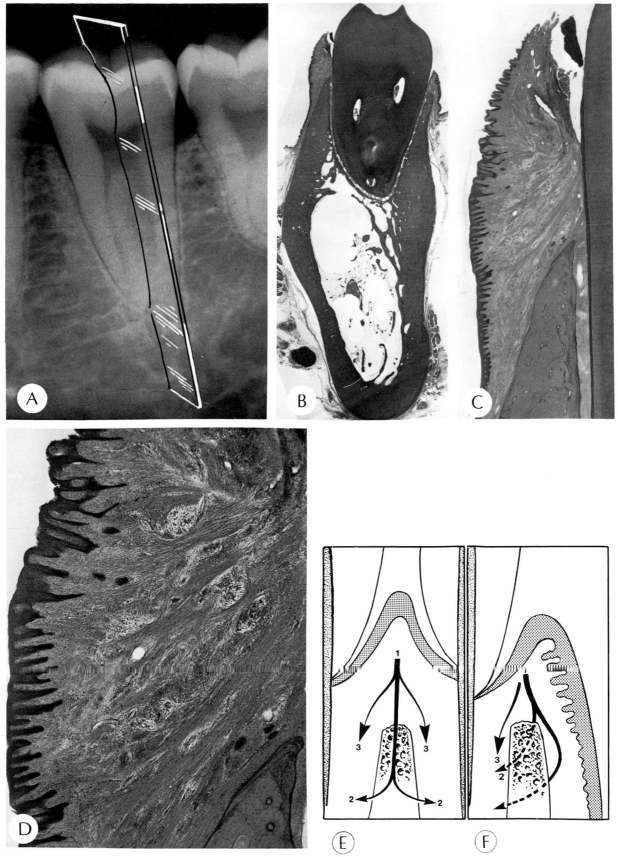

Figure 73

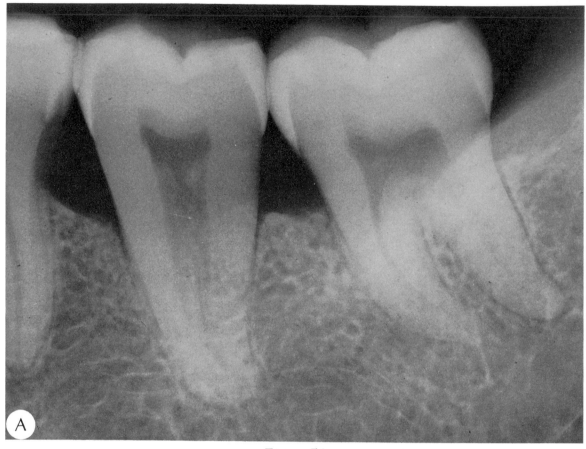

Figure 74

A. Radiograph of mandibular molar area. Note horizontal interdental septum between second and third molars despite different levels of cemento-enamel junctions of approximating teeth. Radiopaque areas in pulp chambers are pulp stones.

See illustrations on opposite page.

PATHWAY OF INFLAMMATION

In periodontal disease the angulation of the crest of the interdental bone does not necessarily follow a line drawn between the adjacent cemento-enamel junctions as it does in periodontal health. Periodontal disease introduces inflammatory and traumatic changes which in addition to causing bone destruction often alter the angulation of the interdental septum.

In the mandibular molar area illustrated here, there is radiographic evidence of bone loss (Fig. 74A). The crest of the interdental septum between the first (left) and second molars is angular approximating a line drawn between the cemento-enamel junctions of the adjacent tooth surfaces. The interdental septum between the second and third molars is horizontal despite the different levels of the cemento-enamel junctions of the approximating teeth (Figs. 74A and B). In periodontal health, the angulation of the bone would expectedly be parallel to a line drawn between the cemento-enamel junctions.

Between the second and third molars, inflammation extends from the gingiva into the center of the interdental septum in the soft tissue around the blood vessels which seems to act as a path of least resistance to the spread of the inflammation (Figs. 74B and C).

Between the first and second molars the bone is angulated approximately parallel to a line drawn between the adjacent cemento-enamel junctions. There is calculus, gingival inflammation, periodontal pockets and bone loss, and the interdental crest is reduced in height and concave.

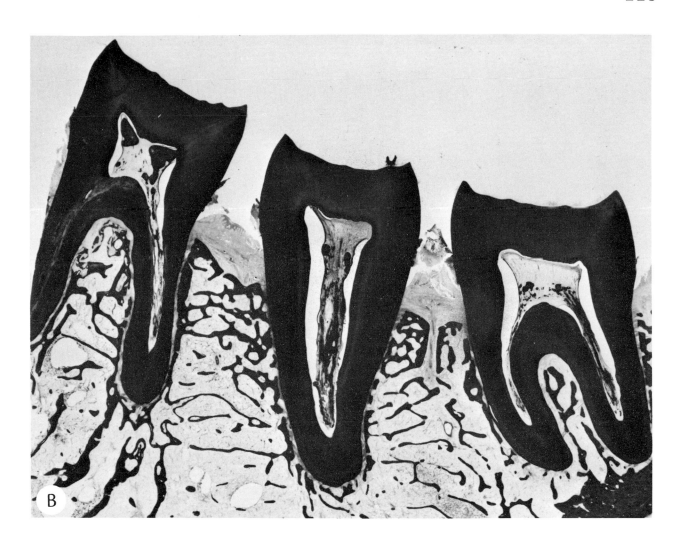

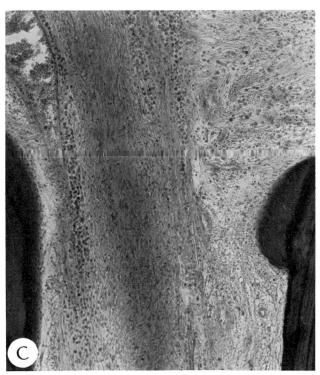

Figure 74

Legend continued.

B. Survey mesio-distal section of mandibular area shown in A. There is horizontal bone loss between the second and third molars despite different levels of cemento-enamel junctions. The inflammation extends from the gingiva into the center of the interdental septum following the path of the blood vessels. Calculus and periodontal pockets are present in relation to all three molars. Note pulp stones (compare with A).

C. High power of interdental area between second and third molars shown in B. Note channeling of leukocytes along blood vessel directly into crest of bone.

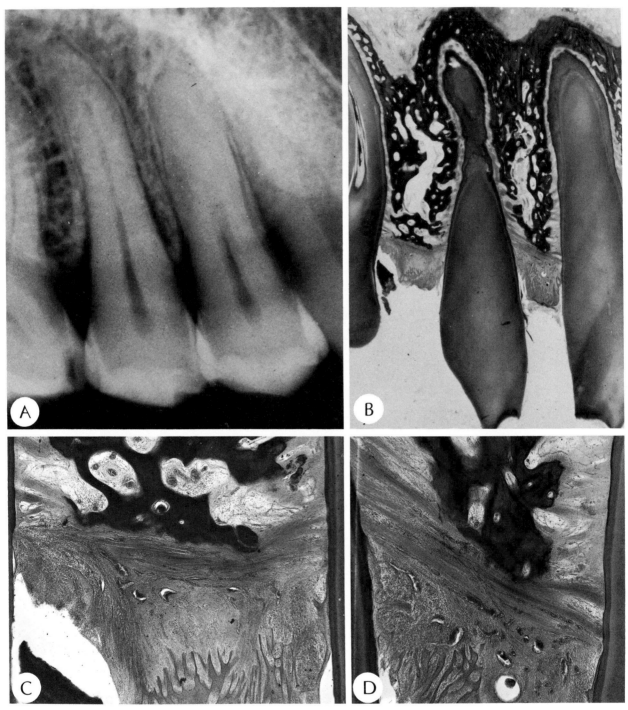

Figure 75

A. Radiograph of maxillary premolar area. Note wedge-shaped thickening of periodontal space in the coronal third of the root mesial and distal to the second premolar (left).

B. Survey mesio-distal section of premolar area shown in A. Calculus and periodontal pockets are present on first and second premolar and molar roots and there is reduction in the height of the alveolar bone. The interdental gingival papillae are inflamed.

See illustration on opposite page.

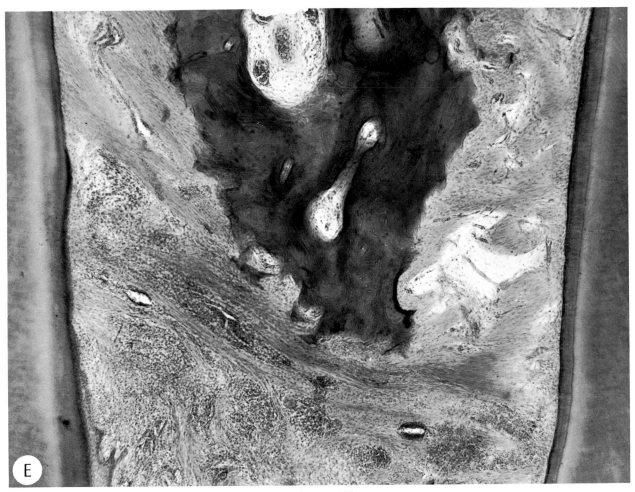

Figure 75

Legend continued.

C. Higher power of the interdental area distal to the second premolar (center) shown in B. The transseptal fibers extend horizontally across the crest of the bone and perpendicular to the premolar and molar tooth surfaces. The alignment of the periodontal ligament fibers between the bone and the roots is normal. Inflammation extends between the transseptal fibers.

D. Higher power of the interdental area mesial to the second premolar (center) shown in B. The transseptal and the deeper periodontal ligament fibers on the mesial surface of the second premolar (left) are oblique and angulated in an apical direction, suggesting a compressive mesial force. Inflammation extends from the gingiva directly into the periodontal ligament. Distal to the first premolar (right), the periodontal ligament fibers are distended and perpendicular to the root and interdental septum.

On the mesial surface of the second premolar in the coronal third, the periodontal ligament is widened and wedge-shaped when compared with the periodontal ligament distal to the first premolar. The epithelial attachment at the base of the pocket on the second premolar is located further apically than the base of the pocket on the first premolar. The interdental bone is reduced in height and presents an angular crestal defect mesial to the second premolar. Inflammation extends from the gingiva to the transseptal fibers and along the fibers into the periodontal ligament.

E. Section taken from the same tissue block as that shown in D. The transseptal fibers are perpendicular to the first premolar root (right) but angulated and parallel to fibers deeper in the periodontal ligament mesial to the second premolar (left). Inflammation extends along the altered transseptal fibers directly into the periodontal ligament. Note osteoclastic resorption along the angular bone surface.

The first and second premolars are erupted to a comparable occlusal level. The angular defect on the mesial aspect of the second premolar is therefore not attributable to differences in the levels of the approximately cementoenamel junctions.

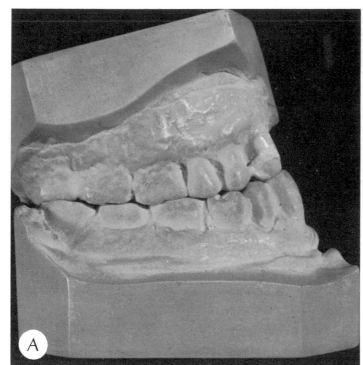

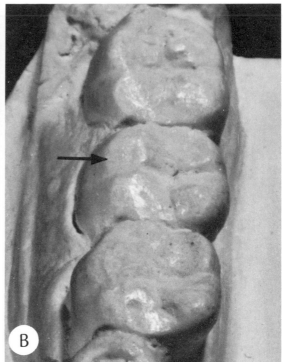

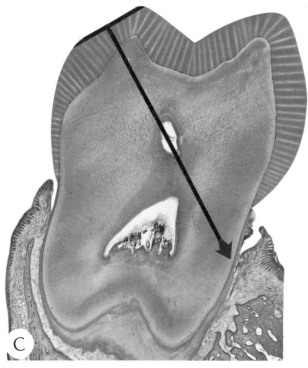

Figure 76

A and *B.* Study cast of mandibular molar and premolar area showing facets at the facio-occlusal angle of the molar and second premolar teeth. Arrow (B) indicates area from which tissue section (C) was taken.

C. Facio-lingual section of mandibular second molar showing pocket formation on facial (left) and lingual (right) surfaces. The flat black line on the enamel outlines the facet and the arrow indicates the direction of the occlusal forces suggested by the facet.

See illustrations on opposite page.

D. Higher power of the facial surface of C showing well formed periodontal ligament fibers extending from the crest of the bone to the cementum. Inflammation from the marginal gingiva extends lateral to the crestal fibers and external to the bony plate.

E. Higher power of the lingual surface of C showing inflammation extending directly into the periodontal ligament. Excessive occlusal pressure is suggested by compression and oblique direction of periodontal ligament fibers apical to widened funnel-shaped area (arrow) produced by angular bone loss.

F. Higher power of periodontal ligament and alveolar crest shown in D. The crestal bone is being resorbed on both the internal and external surfaces. The periodontal ligament fibers are elongated and the inflammation extends over the external bone surface. Note Haversian system in center of lamellated bone.

G. Higher power of periodontal ligament and crest of bone shown in E. The fibers are compressed and seem to be taking on an amorphous appearance. They are surrounded by the inflammatory infiltrate. The coronal bone tip projecting into the periodontal ligament is undergoing osteoclastic resorption.

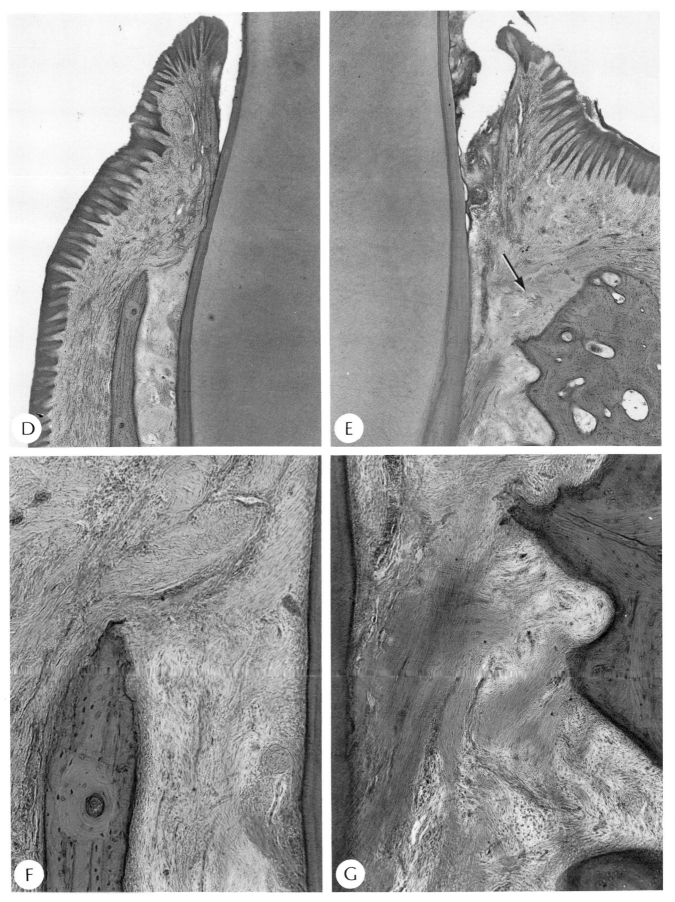

Figure 76

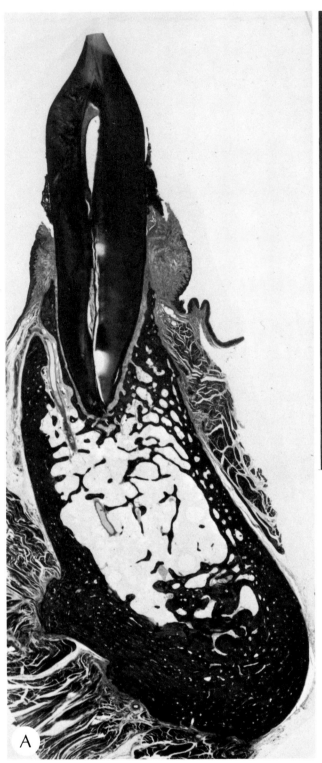

Figure 77

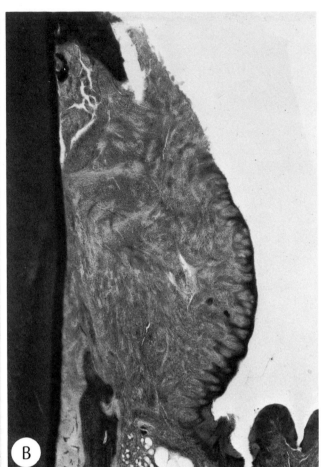

See legend on opposite page.

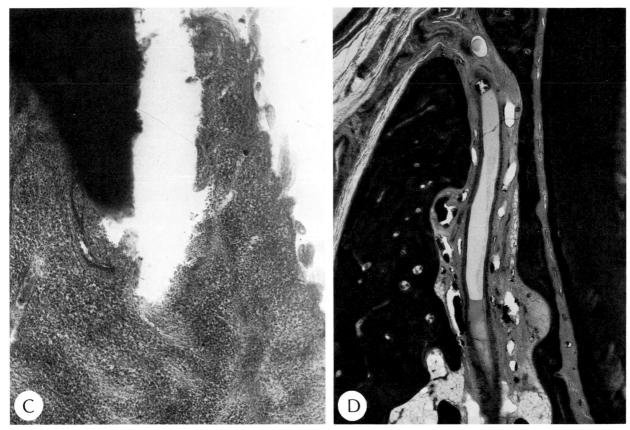

Figure 77

A. Facio-lingual section of mandible and incisor tooth. On the buccal (right) there are heavy deposits of calculus that impinge on the enlarged, inflamed gingiva. The bone height on the buccal is considerably reduced. The dense cortical plates which comprise the outer portion of the mandible are thicker at the base. The curvature to the right forms the prominence of the chin (mental protuberance). The small bony masses on the lower portion of the lingual (left) cortical plate are the mental spines (genial tubercles) from which the genioglossus and geniohyoid muscles arise. There is reduction in the height of the lingual alveolar bone and a large vessel enters the jaw in this area. The calculus on the lingual does not impinge on the gingiva, which is less inflamed and not as enlarged as on the buccal.

B. Facial aspect of mandibular incisor illustrated in A. The inflamed gingiva is enlarged and heavily infiltrated with leukocytes. There is degeneration of collagen fibers and resorption of bone. Note penetration of calculus into the tissue.

C. Higher power of crest of labial gingiva and calculus seen in B. There is severe inflammation, degeneration, necrosis and ulceration of tissue adjacent to the calculus. Note extremely dense leukocytic infiltrate in this area.

D. Higher power of vessel entering the jaw shown in A. Numerous smaller vessels are present in the periodontal ligament and in the connective tissue around the large vessel.

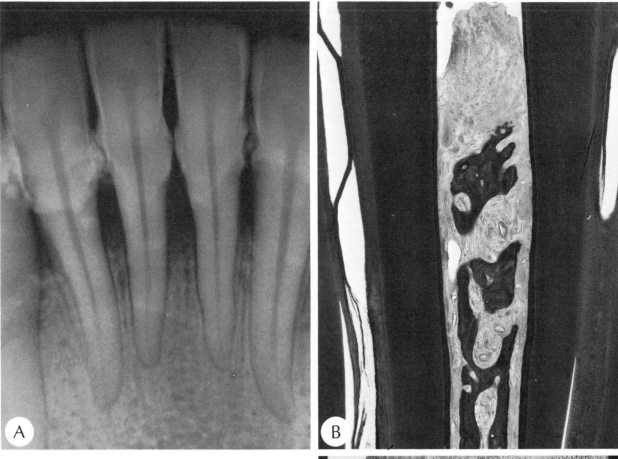

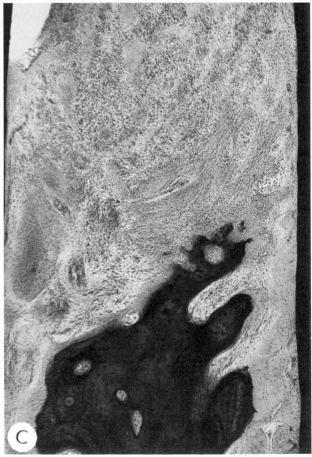

Figure 78

A. Radiograph of mandibular anterior teeth. There is generalized horizontal reduction in bone height. The dark vertical lines seen in the central portion of the interproximal bone represent the nutrient (interdental) canals which contain arterioles. Heavy calculus deposits are noted on all teeth.

B. Interdental area between right central (left) and lateral (right) incisors illustrated in A. The gingiva is inflamed and there is reduction in bone height.

C. Higher power of interdental crestal area shown in B. As a result of inflammation, the collagen fibers are fragmented and undergoing degeneration. Both formation and resorption of bone are seen on the crestal surface. Note relationship of base of periodontal pocket (upper left) to crest of bone.

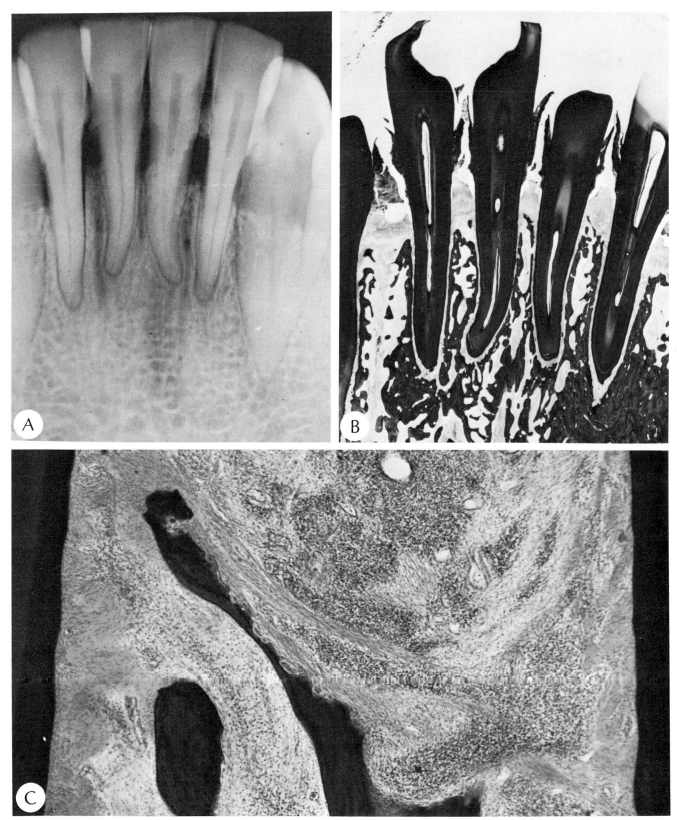

Figure 79

A. Radiograph of mandibular incisor area showing horizontal bone loss. The dark vertical areas in the interdental region represent the nutrient (interdental) canals which contain arterioles. A considerable amount of calculus can be seen on the teeth.

B. Mesio-distal section of mandibular incisor area shown in A. Numerous arterioles can be seen in the interdental bone. Note generalized horizontal bone loss, and heavy deposits of calculus.

C. Higher power of crest of bone in the interdental area between mandibular right central (left) and lateral (right). Inflammation has fragmented the collagen fibers and penetrated into the bone. Numerous Howship's lacunae, containing osteoclasts, are noted on the surface of the resorbing bone.

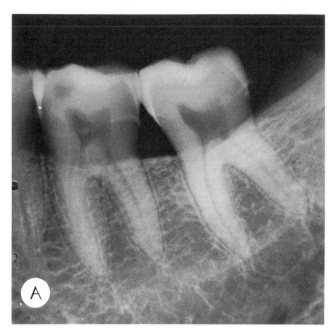

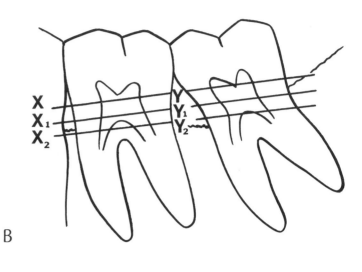

Figure 80

A. Radiograph of mandibular second and third molars. There is generalized horizontal reduction in bone height.

B. Diagram of molar teeth shown in A. The heavy horizontal lines indicate the depth of the planes of sections shown in Figs. 81A, B and C. The letters correspond to the interdental areas shown in the histologic sections on pages 125, 126, 127.

Figure 81.   See illustrations on opposite page.

A. Plane of section represented by line XY shown in Fig. 80B. The plane is through the upper portion of the gingival papillae. At this level, periodontal pockets surround the teeth with the exception of the distal portion of the third molar (right) where there are connective tissue fibers embedded in the tooth.

B. Plane of section represented by line X_1Y_1 shown in Fig. 80B. The periodontal pockets have not descended to this level except for the buccal (top) of the first and second molars and a small area on the mesio-buccal of the third molar. Bone surrounds the posterior portion of the third molar.

C. Plane of section represented by line $X_2 Y_2$ shown in Fig. 80B. The only periodontal pocket to reach this level is seen on the buccal of the second molar. The bone around the third molar has increased and there is some present interdentally between the first and second molars.

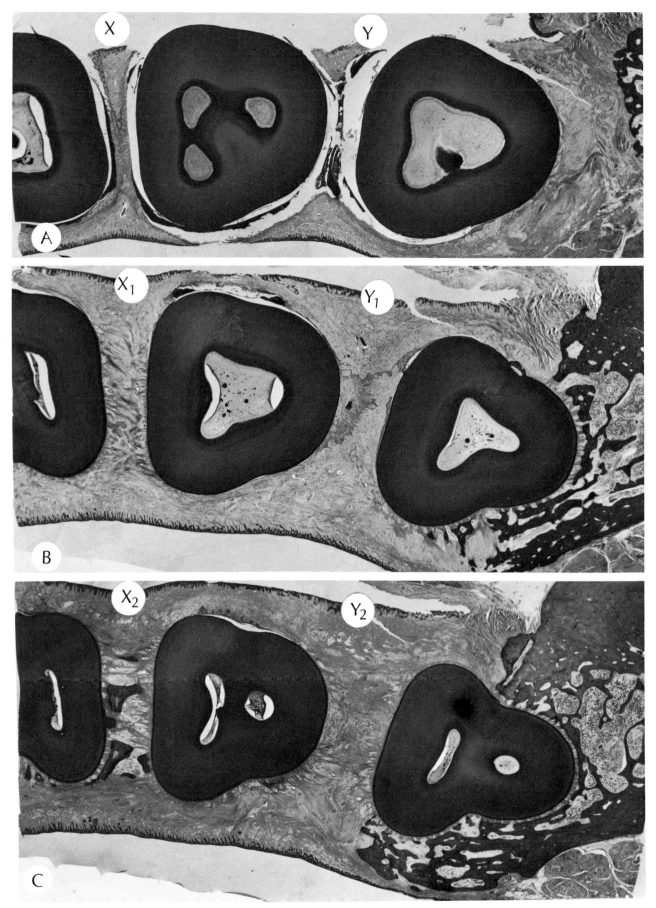

Figure 81

MESIAL MIGRATION

Teeth migrate mesially throughout life. This migration is termed mesial drift and is a normal physiologic occurrence. There are numerous factors which contribute to this mesial movement. These include pressure from the musculature in and about the mouth; chewing; swallowing; axial inclinations of the teeth; cuspal inclinations; growth and eruption patterns; continuous eruption of the teeth and other factors which compensate for tooth wear. Mesial migration combined with continuous eruption helps maintain the interproximal and occlusal contacts of teeth and determines their position in the jaw. As teeth are abraded occlusally, continuous eruption helps compensate for loss in vertical dimension. In like manner, teeth in proximal contact wear in these areas as a result of friction. The interproximal wear tends to broaden the contact area, flatten the proximal surface of the tooth and reduce the antero-posterior length of the dentition. This loss of tooth substance from the proximal region reduces the dental arch about one centimeter during the life of an individual. In addition to the size of the teeth and the space available for them in the dental arch, migration of teeth may be one of the factors involved in tooth crowding which is frequently seen in the anterior region.

As a tooth migrates mesially, changes take place in the supporting periodontal structures on both mesial and distal aspects. The tissues mesial (anterior) to the tooth are in an area of compression and the resulting pressure favors resorption of bone. The alveolus in this region has an irregular surface with numerous small concavities or indentations called Howship's lacunae which result from osteoclastic resorption. Endosteal bone formation is often seen, the additional bone needed to strengthen the alveolus in areas of resorption. The periodontal ligament fibers are compressed and the blood vessels appear round and often engorged. There is little or no apparent effect on the cementum. Conversely, distal to the tooth, the tissues are in an area of tension. The collagen fibers are elongated and straighter and the blood vessels often elliptical in shape. The average width of the periodontal ligament is greater on the distal than on the mesial. Tension favors osteoblastic activity and deposition of bone. In this manner, the alveolus tends to maintain its width. As on the mesial, the cementum appears unaffected.

The pressures and tensions resulting from mesial migration are not continuous or absolutely regular in occurrence. At times, there is pressure on the distal and tension on the mesial. This is evidenced in histologic sections where tissue changes attributed to pressure are found distally and those resulting from tension, mesially. In addition, both types of changes may be found along the same tooth surface.

Figure 84.   See illustrations on opposite page.

A. Horizontal section through mandibular second (left) and third (right) molar roots. Note cancellous or spongy bone surrounding the roots and dense cortical bone on the surface. The marrow spaces contain some hematopoietic tissue.

B. Higher power of mesial aspect of mesial root of third molar seen in A showing bone (left) and adjacent periodontal ligament. Slight compression is apparent in the periodontal ligament with new bone formation occurring on both sides of the alveolus.

C. Higher power of distal aspect of mesial root of third molar seen in A showing bone (right) and adjacent periodontal ligament. The periodontal ligament fibers when compared with those of B are relatively elongated and tense. The bone has numerous incremental lines indicative of prior bone formative activity and a mesial drift.

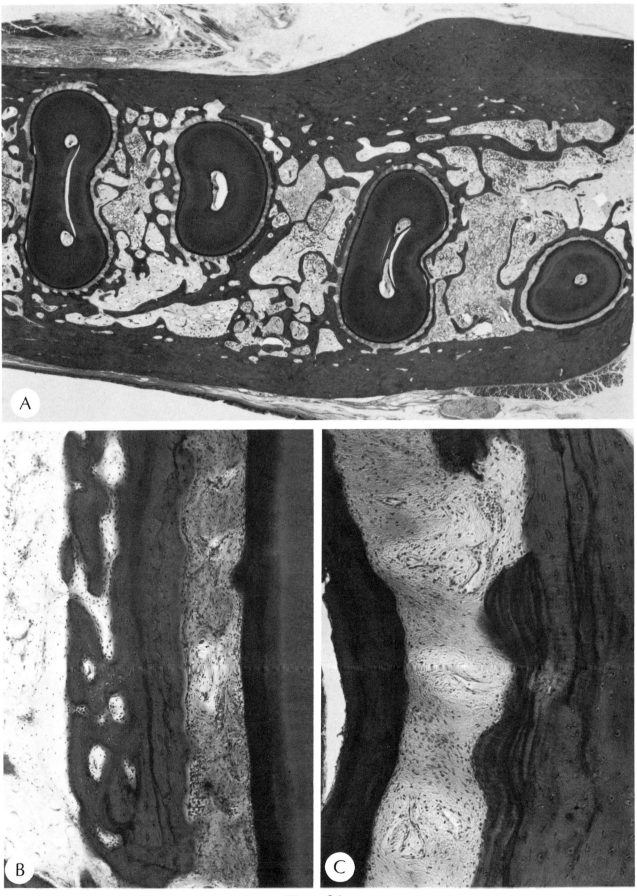

Figure 84

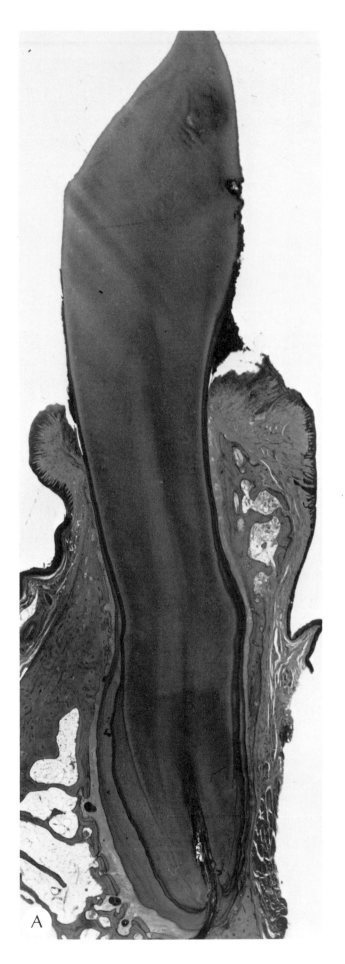

A

Illustration continued on opposite page.

Figure 85

A. Facio-lingual section of mandibular canine. The long axis of the tooth is inclined lingually. In the apical third, the bone is thinned on the facial (right) and thickened on the lingual (left). There has been considerable deposition of cementum in the apical region, particularly on the lingual. The bone height is reduced and the gingiva inflamed.

B. Higher power of lingual crest of bone shown in A. There is compression of the periodontal ligament with necrosis and hyalinization. As a result of compression, the bone at the crest is almost completely resorbed. Only a thin spike of the alveolus remains. The periodontal ligament fibers in this area are being reorganized. More apically, there are other areas of bone resorption adjacent to the compressed periodontal ligament.

C. Higher power of facial crest of bone shown in A. The fibers of the periodontal ligament are extended. New bone is being formed adjacent to the periodontal ligament in response to tension. The distribution of forces on this tooth make it evident that it is being tilted lingually. This results in pressure and resorption of bone lingually at the crest and facially in the apical region. Conversely, there are tension and bone formation lingually, in the apical region and facially, at the crest.

D. Higher power of lingual bone and periodontal ligament in the apical region shown in A. The periodontal ligament fibers are extended and elongated (compare with C). New bone is being formed in this area of tension. Note incremental lines resulting from prior bone deposition.

E. Higher power of facial bone and periodontal ligament in the apical region shown in A. The periodontal ligament fibers are compressed and the normal arrangement of fiber bundles is lacking. Note numerous large osteoclastic cells along scalloped bone margin. The resorption of the bone reduces the pressure and the periodontal ligament is then reorganized. This is a later stage of repair than that seen in B where in some areas the periodontal ligament is still necrotic and hyalinized.

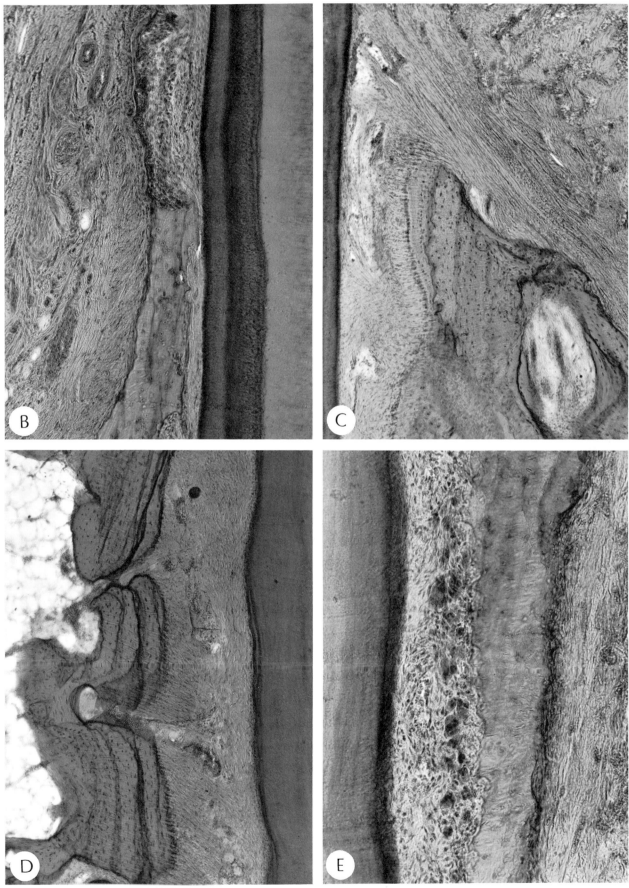

Figure 85

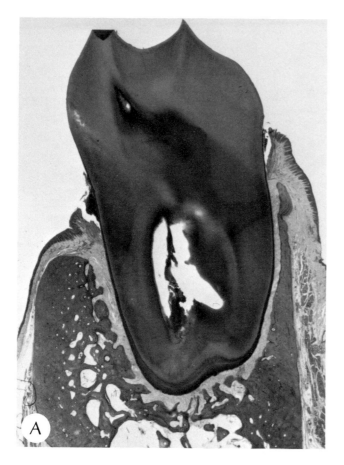

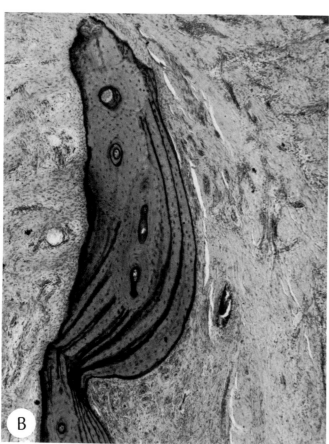

Figure 86

BUTTRESSING BONE

The bone formative activity which occurs in the repair of trauma from occlusion is designated as buttressing bone formation. It represents an attempt to reinforce weakened trabeculae, but it may produce additional effects such as bulbous or ridge-like distortion in the shape of the alveolus and areas of increased radiodensity in the periodontium.

A. Bucco-lingual section through mandibular second molar. On the buccal surface (right) the periodontal ligament is narrow compared with the lingual surface (left). The apical half of the buccal bone surface adjacent to the periodontal ligament is eroded and contains resorption lacunae. This is consistent with persistent pressure buccally.

B. Detailed study of crest of buccal plate shown in A. There is a bulbous cervical ridge formed by prominent peripheral lamellae. The external border of the remainder of the buccal plate consists of bone lamellae separated by deeply staining incremental lines formed in an apparent attempt to buttress the bone against erosion created by buccal pressure. Note osteoclastic resorption at the tip and osteoid and osteoblasts on the external surface.

Figure 87. See illustrations on opposite page.

A. Buccal bone and gingiva prepared with silver stain. This stain is used to bring out detail in collagen fibers and bone and illustrate Sharpey's fibers more clearly.

B. High power of portion of periodontal ligament and bone shown in A. The periodontal ligament fibers are clearly delineated and their embedding in the bundle bone is readily apparent. Bundle bone is defined as that portion of the alveolus which contains Sharpey's fibers. Note how clearly it is demarcated from the more deeply staining bone on the right.

C. Bucco-lingual section of mandibular second molar. There is horizontal bone loss with a suprabony pocket on the lingual (left) and angular bone loss with infrabony pocket on the buccal (right). A pronounced exophytic bone reaction is present in the apical area of the tooth. Both the angular bone loss and osteophytes in the apical region are indicative of increased functional forces.

D. Higher power of buccal alveolar crest seen in C showing angular conformation of bone. A band of collagen fibers runs from the cementum to the crest of the alveolus. The epithelium is migrating apically along the root surface and covers several protruding cemental spikes and a small area of dentin devoid of cementum.

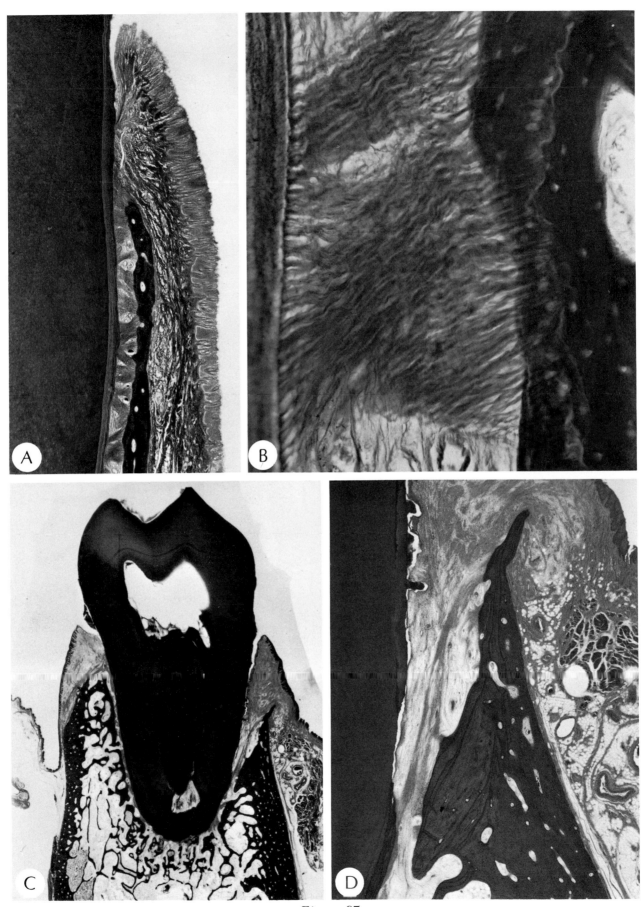

Figure 87

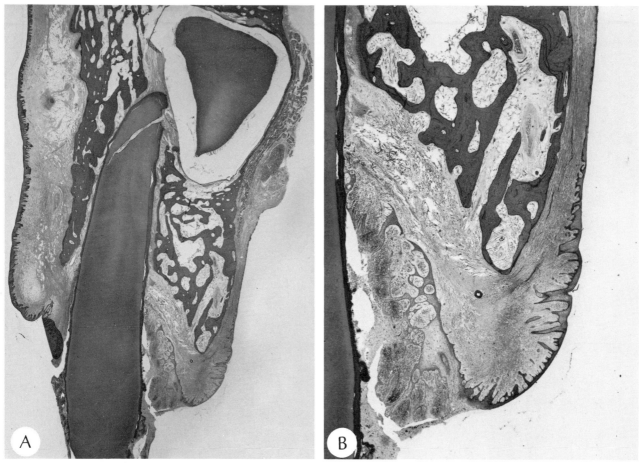

Figure 88

INFRABONY POCKETS

The pathologic changes in infrabony pockets are comparable to those of suprabony pockets. In varied degrees and combinations, inflammation of the pocket wall, suppuration, proliferation and degeneration of the connective tissue and epithelium, and necrosis of the tooth surface are common to all periodontal pockets. However, there is a pattern of bone loss and arrangement of gingival and transseptal fibers which are features peculiar to infrabony pockets.

The pattern of bone destruction associated with infrabony pockets is such that bone loss occurs in a vertical or angular plane rather than horizontally. As a result, it is only beneath the base of the pocket that there is attachment of bone to tooth by periodontal fibers. The surface of the bone which is adjacent and lateral to the pocket wall has no direct connection with the tooth. The "unconnected" bone surface lateral to the soft tissue wall presents a variety of changes which include osteoclastic resorption, repair of previously resorbed areas and areas of inactivity. A comparable variety of bony changes occurs within the alveolar bone along the endosteal surfaces.

In contrast with the lateral bony surface, the bone which is beneath the base of the pocket and is connected to the tooth surface appears to be affected by functional forces as well as by the inflammation in the area.

The arrangement of the gingival and transseptal fibers associated with infrabony pockets stands out when comparison is made with suprabony pockets. In suprabony pockets, the normal arrangement of the gingival and transseptal fibers is maintained by the restoration of new fibers in the area formerly occupied by alveolar bone and periodontal ligament. However, the formation of an infrabony pocket leads to the creation of a new fiber pattern, with an increased length of the gingival fibers and oblique rather than horizontal transseptal fibers. In infrabony pockets located interproximally, fibers extend from the cementum beneath the epithelial attachment along the bony surface up to the crest where they divide into two groups, one of which passes over the crest to the cementum of the adjacent tooth (transseptal); the other extends into the gingival papilla (gingival). In labial and lingual infrabony pockets, one group of fibers extends over the bony crest to become continuous with the fibrous outer periosteum of the bone and the other extends into the gingiva (gingival). The fibers present varying degrees of degeneration and destruction depending upon the extent and severity of inflammatory involvement.

Figure 88

A. Survey section of maxillary lateral incisor showing impacted canine tooth (palatal). Note infra-bony pocket on palatal and incipient infrabony pocket on labial.

B. Higher power of palatal infrabony pocket shown in A. Note the angular pattern of bone destruction and direction of collagen fibers.

C and D. Higher powers of attachment area shown in B. The epithelium is proliferating apically along the root surface. Note angulation of the collagen fibers which follow the contour of the bone and their penetration and destruction by the inflammatory infiltrate.

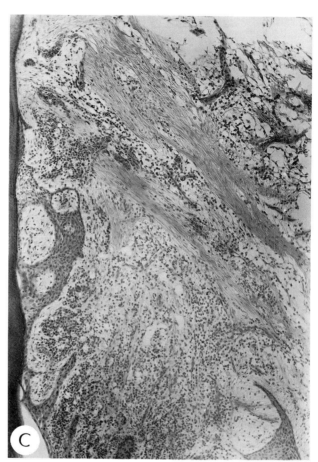

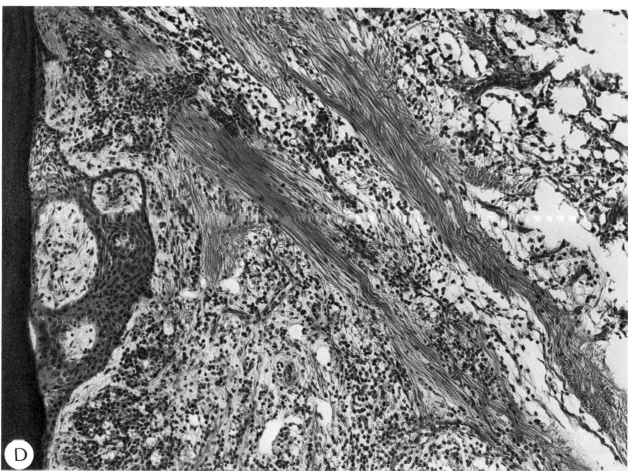

Trauma From Occlusion

It has been demonstrated in experimental animals that trauma from occlusion can alter the pathway of inflammation from the gingiva into the supporting periodontal tissues, modify the pattern of tissue destruction and lead to infrabony pocket formation and angular or vertical bone destruction. It has also been shown that the furcation regions are the areas most susceptible to trauma from occlusion. Similar microscopic findings have been described in human jaws and the observation made that infrabony pockets and angular bone defects in humans can be produced as they have been in animals, by the combined effects of trauma from occlusion and inflammation.

Infrabony pockets and angular osseous defects are not necessarily pathognomonic of the combined effects of inflammation and trauma from occlusion. They may be produced by other factors but as yet the research to determine what these other factors may be has not been done. The possibility that trauma from occlusion combined with inflammation is the responsible etiologic factor must always be considered when infrabony pockets and angular osseous defects occur. Although not infallible and subject to technically created artifacts, radiographs can be very helpful in locating occlusal forces that are destructive to the periodontium. The presence of angular osseous defects on the radiograph may not always mean trauma from occlusion, but it is strongly suggestive. No other local factors have been so consistently identified with angular defects.

The possibility of the existence of trauma from occlusion and periodontal inflammation without infrabony pockets and osseous defects should not be excluded. However, when the latter lesions are present the former etiologic agents must be considered. Conversely, the absence of infrabony pockets and angular osseous defects in periodontitis does not rule out the presence of trauma from occlusion. The combination of inflammation and trauma from occlusion may not have attained sufficient severity to produce such lesions or the anatomy of the teeth and supporting bone may not be conducive to their formation. In such instances the pockets are suprabony and the bone loss is horizontal. Because of the varied combinations of inflammation and trauma from occlusion, angular bone loss may occur beneath suprabony pockets.

Trauma from occlusion per se does not cause any type of periodontal pocket. Local irritation is required to initiate the inflammatory changes leading to periodontal pocket formation. The alterations produced by trauma from occlusion in the supporting periodontal tissues facilitate the development of infrabony pockets, provided there is sufficient local irritation to initiate the process of pocket formation. Trauma from occlusion may also produce angular widening of the crestal bone without periodontal pockets in the absence of local irritants severe enough to cause pockets.

Trauma from occlusion is reversible. Under proper conditions the tissue injury produced by excessive occlusal forces undergoes repair. For example, occlusal forces may be diminished by teeth moving from the offending occlusal antagonists. In a broad sense, trauma from occlusion may be considered to be tissue injury plus a series of changes, whereby the periodontium attempts to adapt to excessive occlusal forces. In attempting repair, the periodontium may undergo morphologic changes such as pronounced widening of the periodontal ligament and resorption of the adjacent bone. These changes cushion the impact of the offending occlusal forces so that the forces are no longer injurious to the altered periodontium, but may also result in loosening of the teeth. The fact that trauma from occlusion is potentially a reversible change does not minimize its importance in periodontitis. The responsible excessive forces must be eliminated in order to allow reversal of the periodontal injury to occur.

Figure 90.   See illustrations on opposite page.

A. Radiograph of mandibular premolar area. The first premolar (left) shows widening of the periodontal ligament space at the crest and angular conformation of the bone. Note reduction in bone height around both teeth.

B. Mesio-distal section of premolar area shown in A. There are infrabony pockets and angular bone loss mesial and distal to the first premolar (center). The second premolar (right) has suprabony pockets. The gingival papillae are inflamed and there is reduction in bone height.

C. Higher power of crest of bone between first premolar (left) and second premolar (right) shown in B. The inflammation is concentrated laterally and apically to the pocket and is being channeled directly into the periodontal ligament distal to the first premolar. The alveolar crest fibers mesial to the second premolar are elongated and tense and new bone is being formed in this area.

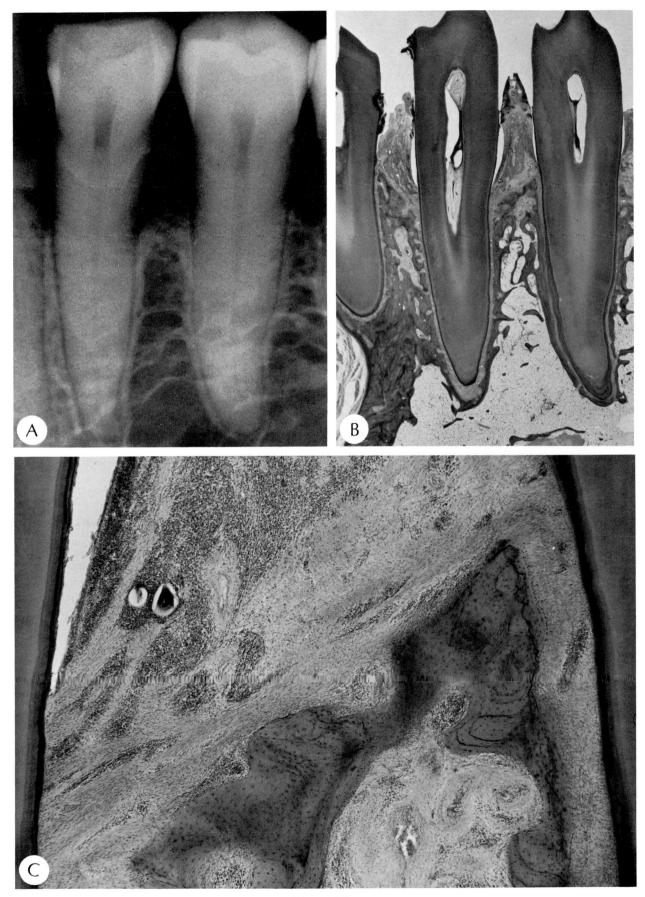

Figure 90

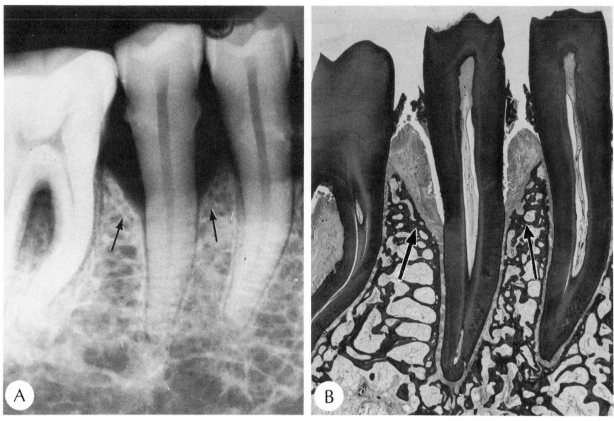

Figure 91

A. Radiograph of mandibular premolar area showing angular osseous defects mesial and distal to the second premolar (arrows) and bifurcation involvement in the first molar.

B. Mesio-distal section of premolar area shown in A. Note infrabony pockets and osseous defects (arrows) on the mesial and distal surfaces of the second premolar. There is considerable loss of tissue in the bifurcation area.

TRAUMA FROM OCCLUSION

Trauma from occlusion occurs in three stages. The first stage is injury to the periodontium. The second is repair of the injured tissues in an effort to restore the periodontal structures to normal. If the force persists and repair is not successful, the third stage is reached. It consists of alterations in the morphology of the periodontium to adapt to the occlusal forces. This includes widening of the periodontal ligament which is most pronounced in the coronal half of the periodontium accompanied by angular resorption of the bone. The periodontal ligament is widened in an effort to cushion the tooth against the force. When it becomes sufficiently widened so that the force is alleviated a state of equilibrium is reached and the force is no longer injurious. A change in the morphology of the periodontium is the result.

See illustrations on opposite page.

C. Higher power beneath infrabony pocket on the distal surface of the second premolar seen in Fig. 91B, showing remodeling of the bone with funnel-shaped widening of the periodontal ligament. Note inflammation in the periodontal ligament.

D. Higher power beneath infrabony pocket on the mesial surface seen in B. As in C, there is remodeling of the bone with funnel-shaped widening of the periodontal ligament.

E. Detailed view of the distal crestal bone area seen in C showing resorption along the margin of the bone. There is resorption of lamellar bone which is being replaced by concentric lamellae around the marrow space. Note that the concentric lamellae are also undergoing resorption.

F. Detailed view of the mesial crestal bone area seen in D, showing inflammation at the crest of the bone and deeper in the periodontal ligament. Note resorption of a portion of the spherical lamella.

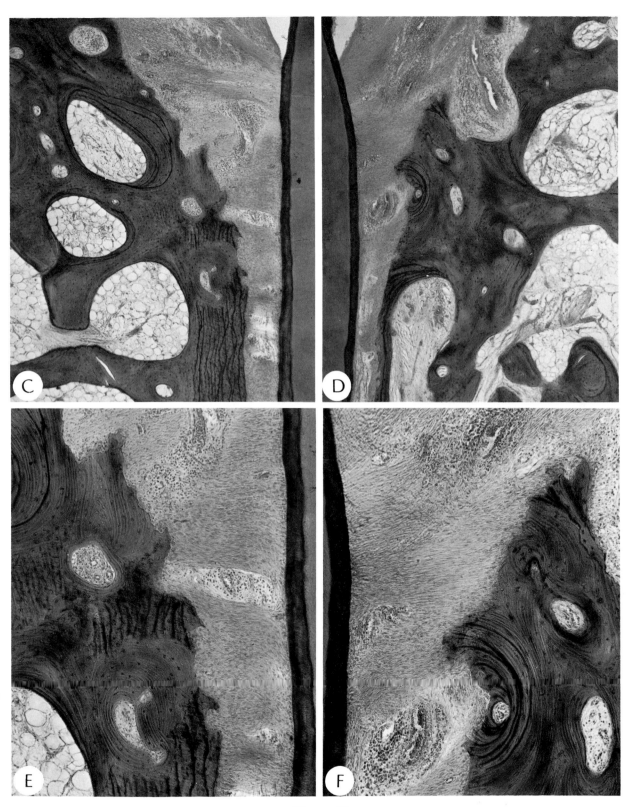

Figure 91

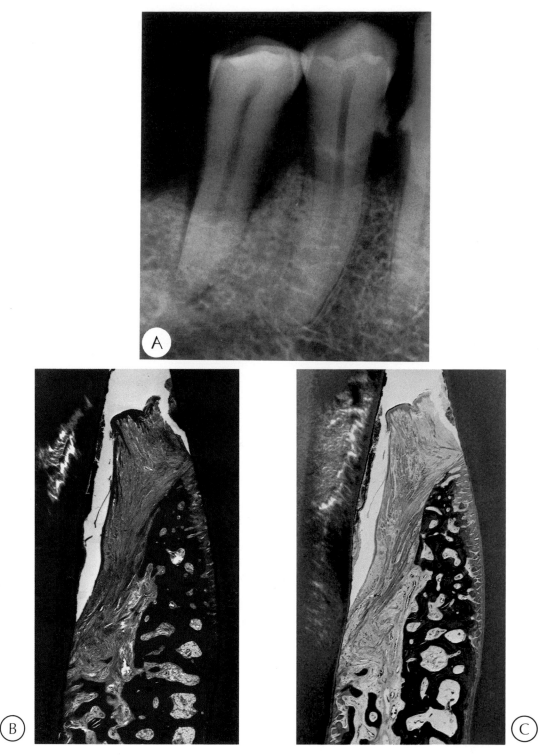

Figure 92

A. Radiograph of mandibular canine and premolar area. There is angular reduction in bone height mesial to the second premolar (left). The angulation of the bone between the canine (right) and first premolar (center) which is seen histologically is not readily apparent radiographically. Several spicules of calculus are adherent to the teeth.

B. Higher power of interdental area between the premolar teeth shown in Fig. 93A. The crest of bone supports only the distal of the first premolar as the infrabony pocket intervenes between the bone and the tooth on the mesial of the second premolar. Because the coronal portion of the septum supports only one tooth it is classified as a hemiseptum. The transseptal fibers are angulated and follow the contour of the bone.

C. Higher power of interdental area between first and second premolars shown in Fig. 93B. The Mallory Connective Tissue stain used in this section depicts clearly the angulated transseptal and remaining gingival fibers. Note difference in height of attachment of periodontal ligament fibers distal to first premolar (right) and mesial to second premolar (left).

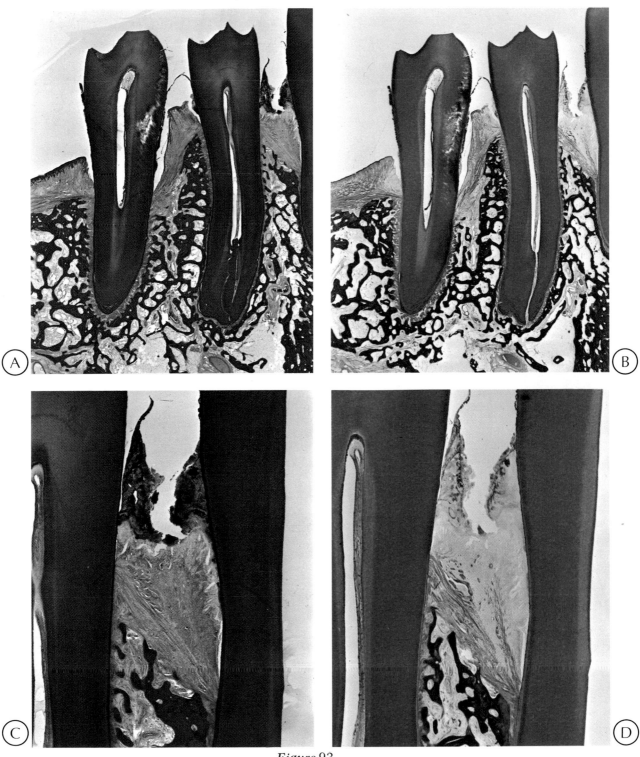

Figure 93

A. Mesio-distal section of mandibular premolar and canine teeth shown in Fig. 92A. There are infrabony pockets and angular bone loss mesial to the second premolar (left) and distal to the canine (right). Suprabony pockets with horizontal bone loss are seen distal to the second premolar and mesial and distal to the first premolar.

B. Section taken from same tissue block as that shown in A and stained with Mallory's Connective Tissue stain to demonstrate collagen fibers. In areas of the gingiva where the inflammation is heaviest such as between the canine and first premolar and distal to the second premolar the collagen fibers are totally destroyed.

C. Higher power of interdental area between the canine and first premolar teeth shown in (A). A considerable amount of calculus is present as well as a dense leukocytic infiltration in the gingiva. Note angulation of transseptal fibers and bone.

D. Higher power of crestal interdental region between the canine and first premolar teeth shown in (B). Note that the gingival fibers are almost totally destroyed by the inflammatory disease. The transseptal fibers are a more constant finding than the other gingival fibers and are usually seen even in the presence of relatively severe inflammation. They are, however, fragmented and less dense than normal.

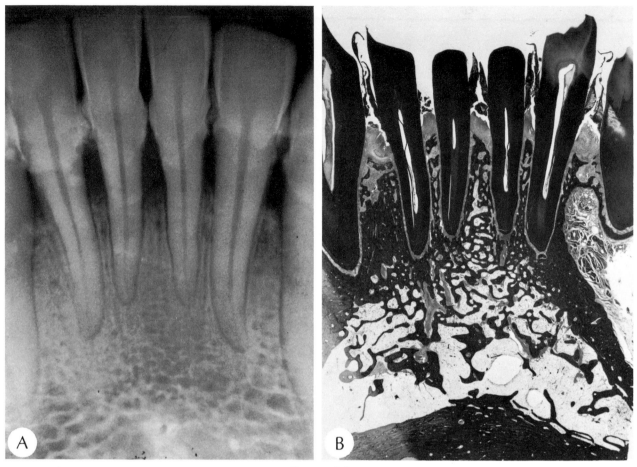

Figure 94

A. Radiograph of mandibular anterior region showing generalized alveolar bone destruction with linear widening of the periodontal ligament space mesial to the right canine (right). Note calculus deposits on all teeth.

B. Mesio-distal section of mandibular anterior region shown in A. There is generalized gingival inflammation with periodontal pocket formation and bone destruction. Calculus deposits are adherent to all teeth. The periodontal ligament on the mesial surface of the right canine (right) is widened as suggested by the radiograph. There are interspersed small bone trabeculae not apparent radiographically and an angular defect on the mesial surface of the right central incisor, for which there is no radiographic indication.

Illustrations continued on opposite page.

TRAUMA FROM OCCLUSION

In this case, the mesial aspect of the canine was subjected to trauma from occlusion as indicated by the changes in the periodontal ligament and bone. Inflammation extended directly into the altered periodontal ligament. The combined result was resorption of bone in the occlusal half of the periodontium with widening of the periodontal ligament, revealed radiographically as a linear thickening of the periodontal ligament space. The periodontal tissues adjacent to the distal surface of the lateral incisor were uninvolved with the traumatic changes. This is evidenced by the fact that the periodontal ligament in this region has a relatively normal fiber bundle arrangement and the adjacent bone surface is not undergoing any extensive resorption.

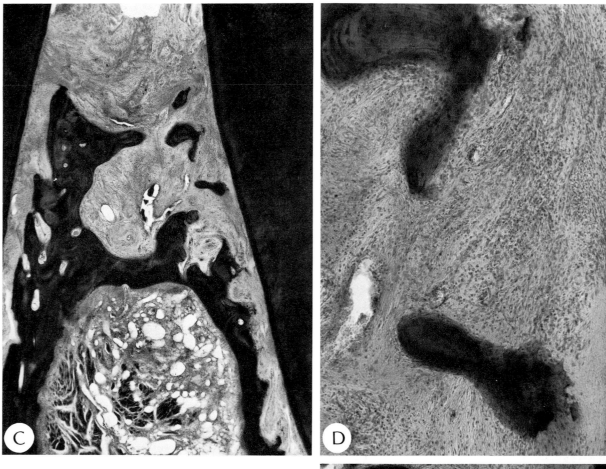

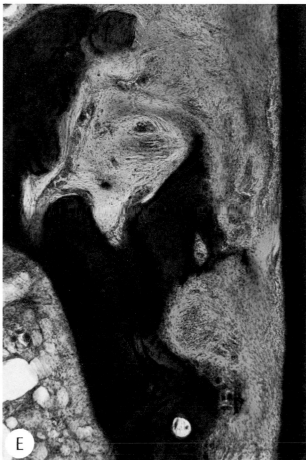

Legend continued.

C. Higher power of interdental area between the right canine (right) and lateral incisor (left) shown in B. In the occlusal half, on the mesial surface of the canine, instead of the dense bone normally present adjacent to the periodontal ligament, the periodontal ligament is widened with interspersed small trabeculae of cancellous bone.

D. Higher power of bone spicules mesial to the canine shown in C. The is compression of the periodontal ligament fibers with a dense leukocytic infiltration. Between the lower bone spicule and the tooth the periodontal ligament is necrotic and hyalinized as a result of excessive compressive forces.

E. Higher power of bone and periodontal ligament shown in C just apical to that seen in D. The regular fiber bundle arrangement is altered with the periodontal ligament fibers more parallel to the tooth surface. Zones of necrosis are present. There is a diffuse leukocytic infiltration extending into the periodontal ligament and osteoclastic resorption and bone formation along adjacent bone surfaces. These changes are consistent with trauma from occlusion.

Figure 94

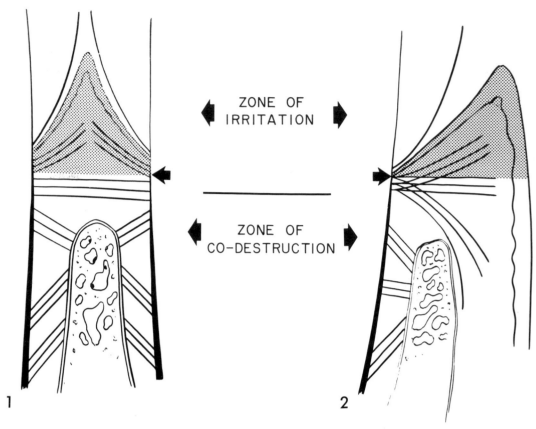

Figure 95

Diagram showing the Zone of Irritation and Zone of Co-destruction in periodontitis. (1) Interproximal view and (2) Bucco-lingual view.

ZONES OF IRRITATION AND CO-DESTRUCTION

To understand the nature of the destructive process in chronic periodontal disease the periodontium may be considered as comprising two disease zones.

I. THE ZONE OF IRRITATION, which consists of the marginal gingiva and interdental gingival papilla and is bounded by the gingival fibers. Local irritants stimulate inflammation in this zone. Degeneration and necrosis of gingival connective tissue, epithelial ulceration and suppuration are its most severe destructive effects. So far as can be determined, trauma from occlusion affects neither the gingival margin nor the interdental gingival papilla. Therefore, inflammation confined to this zone (gingivitis) is unaffected by occlusal forces.

II. THE ZONE OF CO-DESTRUCTION, which consists of the supporting periodontal tissues, the periodontal ligament, alveolar bone and cementum. This zone begins with the transseptal fibers interproximally and with the alveolar crest fibers labially and lingually. In this zone occlusal forces constantly regulate the condition and morphology of the periodontal ligament and alveolar bone. Here inflammation and trauma from occlusion become co-destructive factors in periodontal disease. When the inflammation reaches this zone (periodontitis) its further spread and resultant destruction come under the influence of occlusal forces. It is in this zone that the biologic implications of occlusal forces in periodontal disease are manifest.

Figure 96.   See illustrations on opposite page.

A. Mesio-distal section of mandibular anterior teeth shown in radiograph in Fig. 94A. The sections on this page were stained with Mallory's Connective Tissue stain to illustrate details in the connective tissue. They are taken from the same tissue block as Fig 94B on page 144.

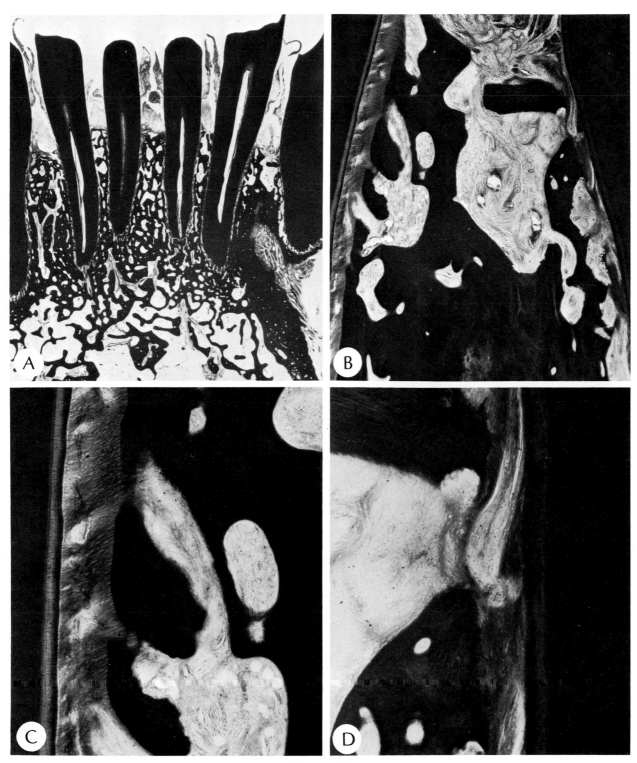

Figure 96

Legend continued.

   B. Higher power of interdental area between the right canine (right) and lateral incisor (left) shown in A. There is compression and bone resorption mesial to the canine resulting from excessive functional forces. The periodontal ligament fibers distal to the lateral incisor are elongated and tense.

   C. Higher power of area distal to the lateral incisor shown in B. As a result of tension in this region the periodontal ligament fibers are elongated. The bundles are well formed and the normal oblique relationship between bone and tooth is apparent.

   D. Higher power of mesial of canine shown in B. Excessive functional force pushes the tooth against the bone. As a result, the fibers of the periodontal ligament are compressed and the normal fiber bundle relationship as illustrated in C is lost. The bone is being resorbed in an attempt to relieve the pressure and allow the tissues in this area to repair.

FURCATION INVOLVEMENT

Furcation involvement is a general term referring to a pathologic condition of the periodontal tissues between the roots of multirooted teeth. When the lesion involves a two-rooted tooth it is called bifurcation involvement; when it is found in a three-rooted tooth, it is termed trifurcation involvement. Lesions in the furcation area are quite common. In a study of human skulls it was reported that about 62 per cent had furcation involvement in one or more teeth. When the ages of the skulls were approximated, it was found that only two had furcation involvement prior to age 30 while more than half showed evidence of this lesion after the age of 60. The teeth most frequently involved with this problem were the maxillary and mandibular first molars.

The etiologic agents related to the development of furcation problems are the same as those involved in the development of periodontitis elsewhere in the mouth. Bifurcation and trifurcation involvement are simply stages in the progression of periodontitis which happens to enter this region of the periodontium. It should be noted, however, that the furcation is the area of the tooth which is most sensitive to occlusal forces. When there is involvement in this region, special attention should be paid to trauma from occlusion as a contributing etiologic agent particularly when there is angular bone loss or a crater-like configuration to the bone.

Sometimes the exposed bifurcation or trifurcation area is not clinically apparent as it may be obscured by the enlarged, inflamed wall of a periodontal pocket. The extent of involvement is determined by exploring the area with a blunt probe. A simultaneous warm blast of air to dry the area and deflect the tissue may also be helpful. The teeth may not be mobile and often present no subjective symptoms such as pain or discomfort. However, there are several possible complications that may occur in furcation involvement. Pain may result from caries or lacunar resorption in the area. Infection may occur in accessory pulp canals which open into the exposed furcation and this may develop into pulpal problems. Food debris may become impacted in the region and result in acute inflammation with gingival or periodontal abscess formation.

To evaluate teeth with furcal involvement, a detailed clinical examination is essential. In the determination of their prognosis, several factors must be considered, such as extent of involvement; amount and contour of remaining bone; mobility of the tooth; relationship of the crown and root to each other and to the adjacent teeth; extent of gingival disease and amount of remaining attached gingiva. One of the most important considerations is the accessibility of the furcation area and the ability and willingness of the patient to cleanse it properly. If the area is adequately maintained, the prognosis of a tooth with furcation involvement should be as good as if not better than a single rooted tooth with the same amount of bone loss because the multirooted tooth has greater anchorage and stability.

Figure 97.   See illustrations on opposite page.

A. Radiograph of mandibular molar area. There is horizontal reduction in bone height and widening of the periodontal ligament space around the roots of the first molar, particularly on the distal. The arrow points to a slight radiolucent area at the crest of the bifurcation of the second molar. An area such as this is indicative of early bifurcation involvement.

B. Bifurcation area of second molar shown in A with arrow pointing to area of tissue loss. There is resorption of bone at the crest and along the distal (right) aspect which is an area of pressure. There is tension on the mesial (left) aspect of the bone with several, clearly delineated, incremental lines indicative of bone formation. The bone is dense and composed of numerous Haversian systems.

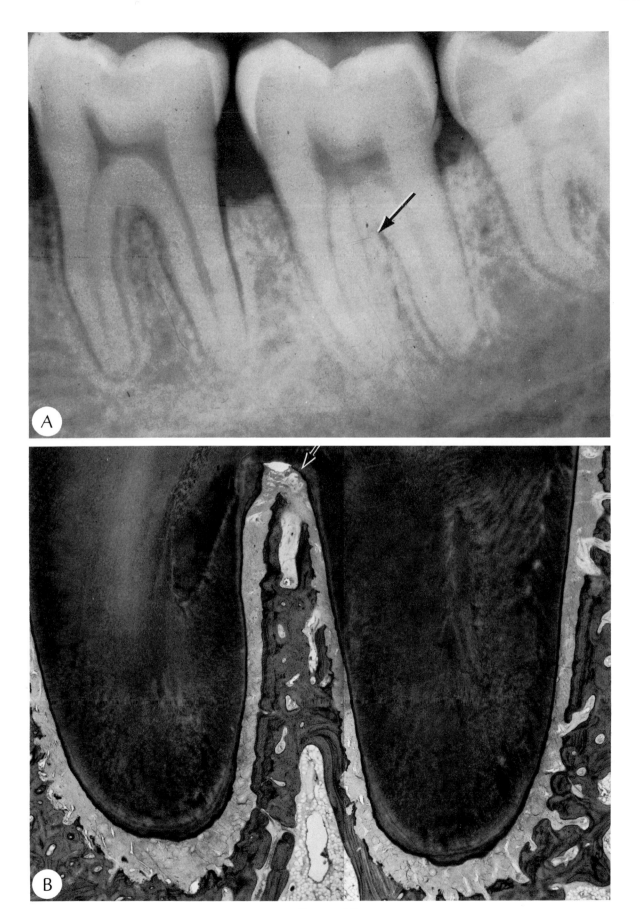

Figure 97

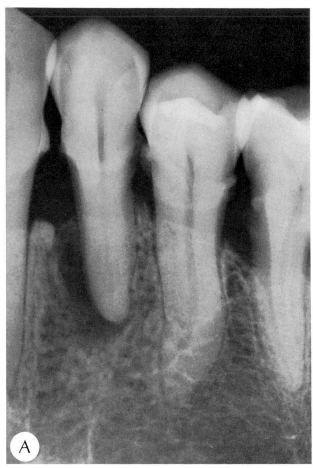

Figure 99

A. Radiograph of mandibular premolar area. A large radiolucent area is present in the mesio-apical region of the first premolar tooth (left). Note absence of caries and presence of heavy calculus deposits.

Figure 99. See illustrations on opposite page.

B. Premolar teeth shown in A. The pocket on the mesial of the first premolar (left) extends beyond the apex. The diagram on the left illustrates this area and shows a probe in the pocket extending to the apical region.

C. Higher power of root of first premolar shown in B. There is considerable debris in the pocket. In this area, the periodontal ligament is totally destroyed and there is no attachment to bone on the mesial. Some fibrotic tissue is noted around the lesion, possibly an attempt at encapsulation.

D. Premolar teeth shown in A from another area of the same tissue block from which B was obtained. The pocket on the mesial extends about one-half of the way down the root surface. The diagram on the left illustrates this area and shows a probe in position (compare with B). Note periapical lesion.

E. Higher power of root of first premolar shown in D. There are some periodontal ligament fibers remaining in the mid-portion of the root attaching the tooth to the bone. Note destruction of tissue around periapical lesion.

PERIODONTAL-PULPAL INTERRELATIONSHIPS

There is a close relationship between the pulp and periodontal tissues. The nerves and vessels which supply the pulp must first pass through the periodontium where they give off branches that help supply the area. An inflammatory or degenerative process involving the blood supply to the periodontal ligament will have an adverse effect on the vascular supply to the pulp. In like manner, factors adversely affecting the pulpal tissue will be detrimental to the periodontal ligament. Direct contamination of the pulp can occur from bacteria and toxic products passing through exposed auxiliary or lateral pulp canals or even through dentinal tubules exposed as a result of periodontal disease. Studies of extracted human teeth have shown that almost 50 per cent had accessory pulp canals. The majority were located in the apical region but a significant number were found in the middle third of the root and in the bifurcation area. Accessory canals need not be directly exposed to the oral fluids for deterioration of the pulp to occur. Toxic products resulting from inflammatory periodontal disease may reach the pulp through these channels while they are still covered with the periodontal tissues. Excessive occlusal forces that are of sufficient magnitude to cause degenerative and necrotic changes in the periodontal tissues are another mechanism which may result in a combined periodontal-endodontic lesion. The resulting toxic products may enter the pulp and lead to degenerative changes. Most often, a pulpal infection is limited to the periapical area where it results in degeneration of the surrounding periodontal tissues. It may, however, reach the surface by forming a fistula which can follow different routes. The inflammation may burrow through the bone and attached gingiva and open directly into the mouth. It may travel coronally through the periodontal ligament and join with inflammation from the gingiva and periodontal tissues that is extending apically. In such cases, there is an additive effect from the combined inflammatory processes which destroys both the pulp and the supporting tissues. The inflammation may extend into a furcation area, break through the attached gingiva and drain into the mouth or it may continue to drain directly from a gingival sulcus.

Pulpal and periodontal tissues are mutually dependent. What is detrimental to one will, in time, adversely affect the other. The degree of pathologic involvement of each tissue and the amount to which each has contributed to a pathologic situation is an important and challenging clinical determination.

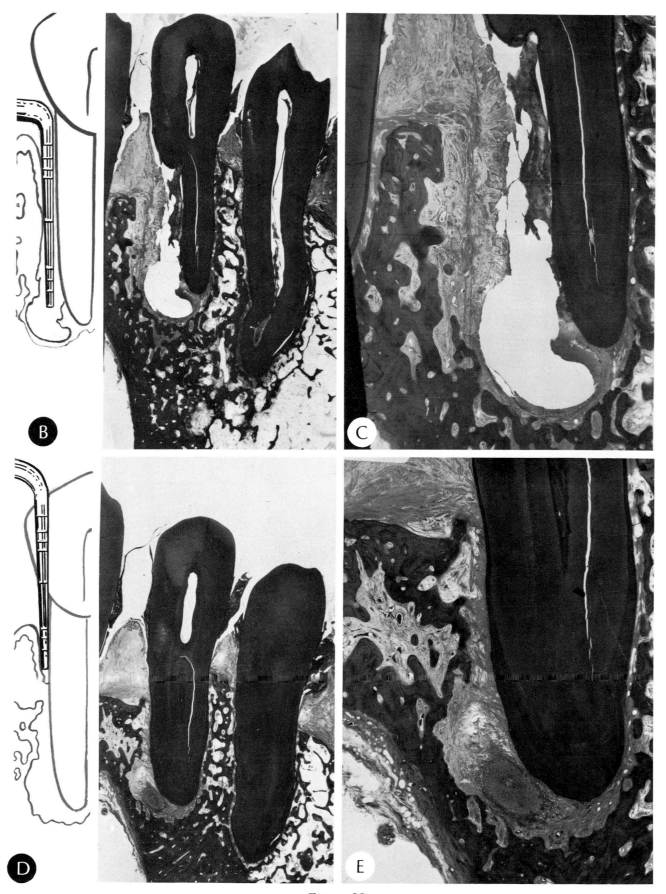

Figure 99

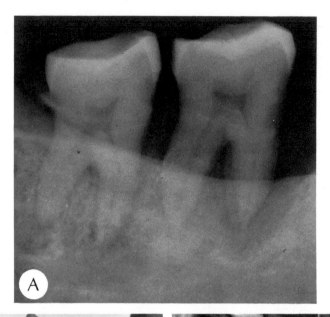

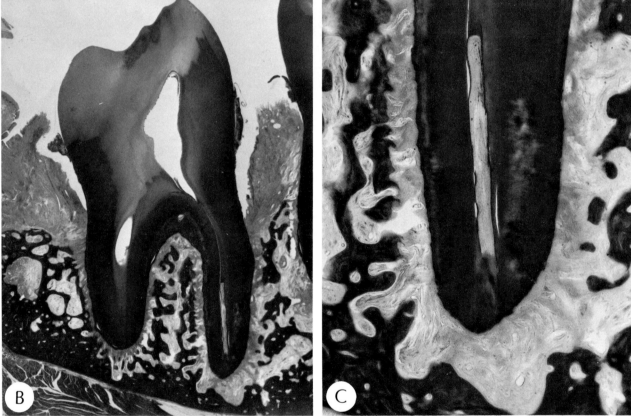

Figure 100

A. Radiograph of mandibular second and third molars. The third molar (left) has generalized bone loss and early bifurcation involvement. The mesial root shows increased width of the periodontal ligament space particularly at the apex. Spurs of calculus are present on the crown. The second molar has more severe bone loss with greater bifurcation involvement. In addition, there are periapical rarefactions about both roots with the mesial root showing erosion and complete loss of surrounding tissue. The radiopaque line distal to the third molar is the external oblique line.

B. Mesio-distal section of third molar seen in A showing considerable reduction in alveolar bone height. There is an infrabony pocket on the mesial, a suprabony pocket on the distal and early bifurcation involvement in the bifurcation area. At the apex of the mesial root, the periodontal ligament is widened.

C. Higher power of mesial root of third molar shown in B. The tissues of the periodontal ligament are degenerating particularly in the apical area.

See illustrations on opposite page.

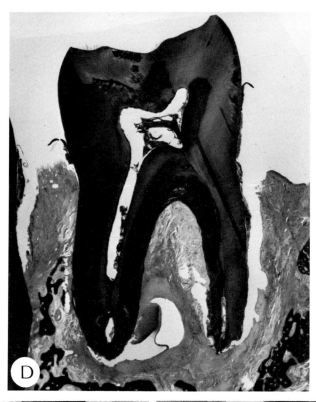

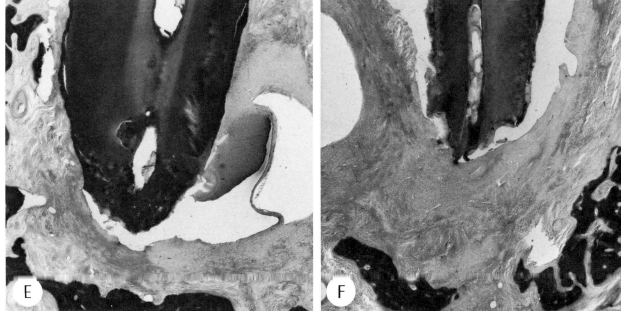

Figure 100

Legend continued.

D. Mesio-distal section of second molar shown in A. With the exception of a small area on the distal portion of the distal root, the periodontal ligament fibers and tooth-supporting bone have been destroyed. Both roots, particularly the mesial, are eroded.

E. Higher power of apical portion of distal root shown in D. There is a well circumscribed cyst-like area about the apex of the root. The periapical inflammatory process is extending coronally in the periodontal ligament. As it advances, it will combine with the inflammatory periodontal lesion, eliminating the remaining tooth-supporting tissues.

F. Higher power of mesial root of second molar shown in D. All of the tissue surrounding the root has been destroyed by the combined effects of the periodontal and periapical lesions. The root surface is severely eroded.

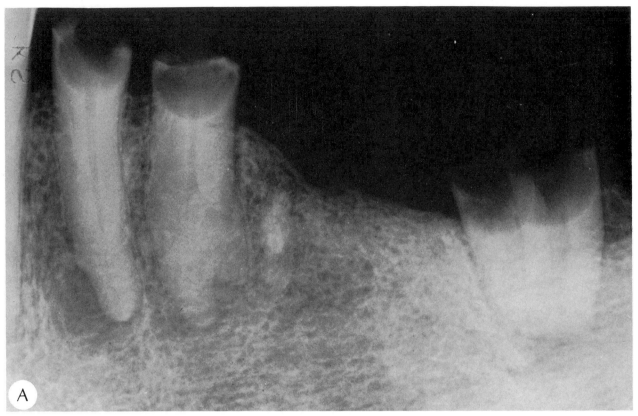

Figure 101

A. Radiograph of mandibular premolar and molar region. The crowns of the teeth have been destroyed. There are radiolucent periapical areas about both premolars. At the apex of the remaining molar there is a radiolucent area surrounded by an area of increased bone density (osteosclerosis). Note the retained root fragment distal to the second premolar.

PERIAPICAL LESIONS

A dental granuloma is a chronic inflammatory lesion located in the periapical region. It usually results from caries and subsequent pulpal infection. The basic histopathologic process is one of chronic inflammation. There are destruction and necro-

(Text continued on page 158.)

Figure 101.   See illustrations on opposite page.

B. Mesio-distal section of mandibular premolar and molar region shown in A. Periapical lesions are present about the roots of all teeth. Note absence of inflammatory reaction around retained root fragment distal to the second premolar.

C. Higher power of premolar roots seen in B. The periapical lesion on the distal of the second premolar (right) has progressed coronally destroying most of the periodontal ligament. At the apex of the first premolar (left), a cystic area is apparent. Note ankylosis of retained root fragment.

D. Higher power of molar root and periapical lesion shown in B. Note proliferation of stratified squamous epithelium at the apex of the root. This lesion would be classified histopathologically as an epithelialed granuloma. The bone surrounding the lesion has become more dense (osteosclerotic). This added bone is a productive response to the inflammatory process.

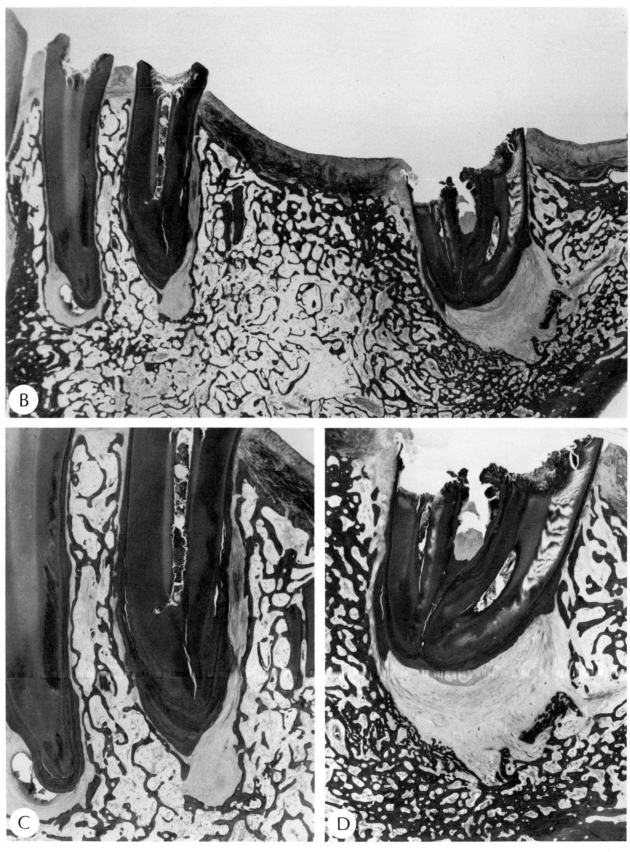

Figure 101

sis of tissue and occasionally cavitation in the central area. The cellular exudate is composed mainly of mononuclear leukocytes such as lymphocytes, plasma cells and histiocytes. Phagocytic cells are active in the removal of the necrotic debris. There are both formation and destruction of bone and fibrous connective tissue. Attempts at repair are seen at the periphery and the lesion may be encapsulated in an effort to limit the spread of the infection. In the area where the lesion is in contact with the tooth the cementum becomes necrotic and will be resorbed. The resorption may continue into the dentin resulting in considerable loss of root structure. Epithelium, which is thought to be derived from the epithelial rests of Malassez, is a common finding in dental granulomas. It sometimes proliferates, forming a network of cells lining all or part of the lesion, which may then be classified as a cyst. Chronic granulomas are usually symptom free and generally found by routine radiographic examination.

Experimental Pathology

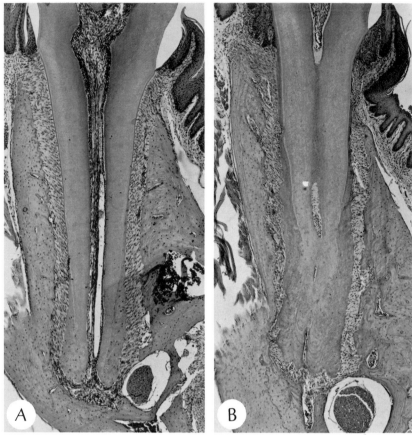

Figure 102

A. Young mouse aged five weeks. Bucco-lingual survey section through first mandibular molar.

B. Old animal aged 14 months. Bucco-lingual survey section through first mandibular molar.

AGE CHANGES IN THE PERIODONTIUM

The mouse is used extensively as an experimental animal in dental research. Because of this, it is important to understand the microscopic appearance of the periodontium of this animal under physiologic conditions, particularly after the teeth have reached their functional antagonists, and as the animals increase in age. Owing to the sparsity of information regarding the physiologic changes in the periodontium of the mouse that occur with age, a microscopic study that would provide this information was undertaken. The investigation revealed that the molars of the albino mouse

(*Text continued on page 162.*)

Figure 102.   See illustrations on opposite page.

C. Detailed study of the crestal area of the buccal plate (left) shown in A. Note sparsity of incremental lines in the bone and reversal line with adjacent new bone formation. Compare thickness of cementum with that in old animal shown in E.

D. Detailed study of the crestal area of the lingual plate (right) illustrated in A showing sparsity of incremental lines compared with lingual plate of old animal shown in F.

E. Detailed study of the crestal area of the buccal plate (left) shown in B. The appositional lines in the bone indicate crestal and buccal increments in conformity with bucco-occlusal tooth eruption.

F. Detailed study of the crestal area of the lingual plate (right) shown in B. The appositional lines in the bone indicate increments at the crest and adjacent to the periodontal ligament in conformity with bucco-occlusal tooth eruption.

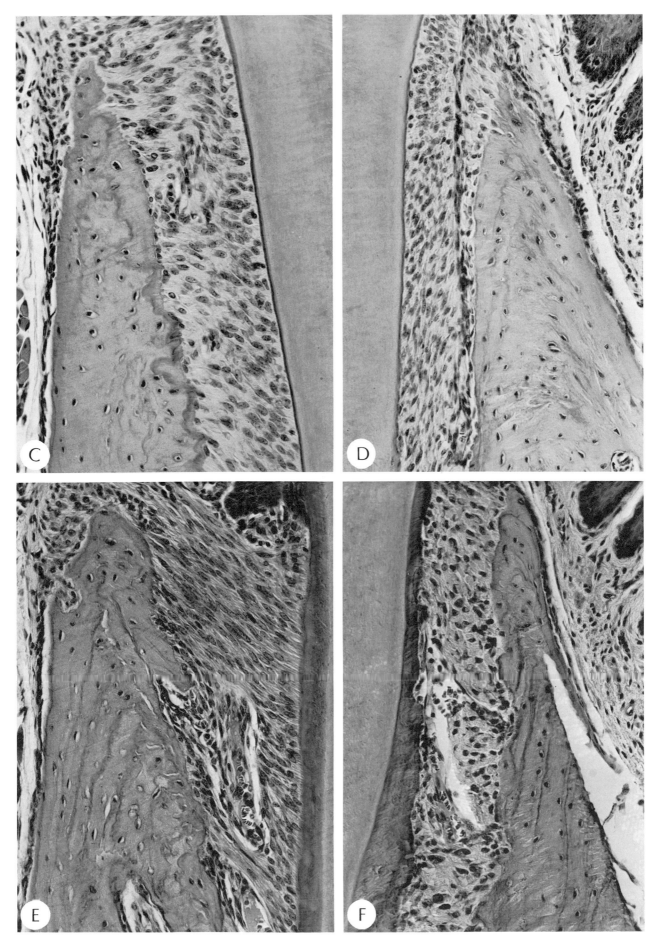

Figure 102

AGE CHANGES IN THE PERIODONTIUM *Continued*

continue to erupt in a bucco-occlusal direction even after contact is made with their functional antagonists. In addition, the tendency to accommodate bucco-occlusal eruption of teeth is of greater consequence than the functional forces in determining the structure and activity of the periodontium. It was determined that the distance between the alveolar crests and the cemento-enamel junction increases with age. This suggests that with age the rate of bone apposition in this area does not keep pace with occlusal eruption of the tooth. Also, with age the mandibular canal tends to be located further apically in relation to the root, since with time the root moves occlusally more than does the canal. The gingival epithelium migrates along the root with increasing age. However, since inflammation is an almost omnipresent finding, it is not possible to determine whether, or to what degree, the initial tendency of the gingival epithelium to migrate along the cementum is attributable to aging or stimulation from local irritation. On the other hand, the proliferative and degenerative tissue changes, pathologic pocket formation, and resorption of underlying bone are so closely related to inflammation in location and severity as to discourage any suggestion that they might be physiologic features of aging.

SYSTEMIC ALTERATION OF ALVEOLAR BONE

There are three basic concepts regarding the nature of bone loss in periodontal disease. The first is that it results solely from an inflammatory process produced by local irritants in the oral cavity. The second is that bone loss in periodontal disease originates as a noninflammatory atrophic degenerative change which is the result of purely systemic influences. The third concept maintains that there are three different types of periodontal disease, the local and systemic types previously mentioned and an additional type which represents a combination of the other two.

Animal experiments were conducted to determine the effect of systemic influences on alveolar bone loss in both the presence and absence of gingival inflammation. In these studies it was shown that the bone of the jaws undergoes changes similar to those which occur in other bones in generalized skeletal disturbances of systemic origin. Alveolar bone loss may, therefore, occur as a result of generalized skeletal disturbances in the absence of gingival inflammation. This is because the height of the interdental septum represents the result of an equilibrium between bone formation and bone resorption. A systemic disturbance which alters this equilibrium by reducing bone formation or increasing bone resorption or both will alter the height of the alveolar bone.

Inflammation in the gingival crevice results in bone resorption and reduction in the height of the interdental septum in the absence of generalized skeletal disturbance. However, the severity of bone loss subjacent to gingival inflammation is increased by generalized skeletal disturbances of systemic origin. Systemic influences may initiate alveolar bone loss or complicate bone loss caused by local factors.

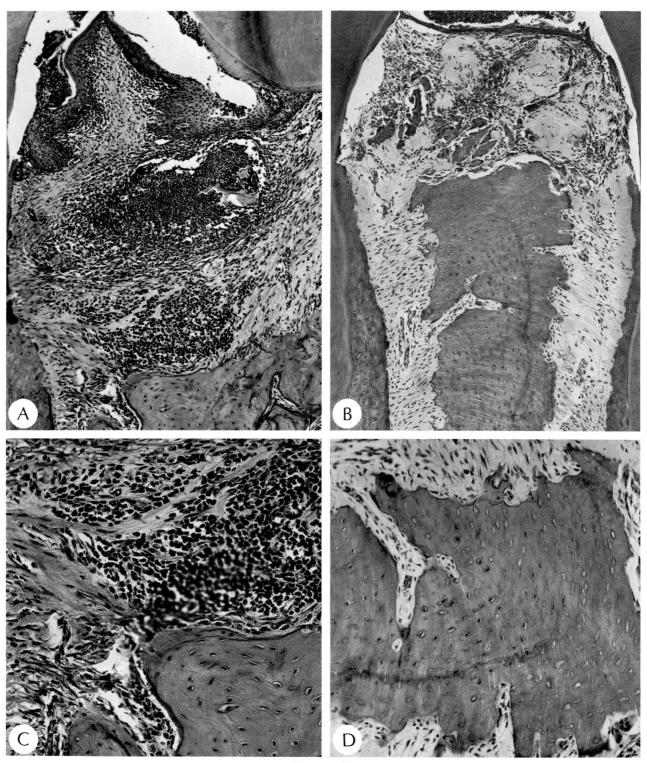

Figure 103

A. Artificially induced gingival inflammation in an animal on a normal diet showing infiltration of lymphocytes to the crest of the interdental septum. (The accumulation of polymorphonuclear leukocytes immediately below the gingival epithelium is a reaction to the presence of a small bone fragment).

B. The effects of starvation on the interdental septum subjacent to an area of artificially induced inflammation showing chronic inflammation in the connective tissue above the bone margin. There is an absence of bone formation in relation to the entire septum.

C. Detail of A. Interdental septum beneath artificially induced gingival inflammation showing lacunar resorption adjacent to osteoblasts and new bone matrix. The underlying bone appears unaltered.

D. Detail of B. Interdental septum beneath area of artificially induced inflammation. There is lacunar resorption along the entire crest with no evidence of bone formation. For a considerable depth below the margin, the lacunae are enlarged and devoid of osteocytes. Fragments of bone are seen in the connective tissue.

Vitamin C Deficiency

Because vitamin C deficiency is a potential factor in the etiology of periodontal disease, it is important that the nature of its influence be established. Vitamin C deficiency alters the response of the periodontal tissues so that the destructive effects of inflammation are accentuated. This exaggerated destruction in the presence of inflammation results partly from an inability to marshal a defensive delimitative reaction to the inflammation and partly from destructive tendencies caused by the deficiency even in the absence of inflammation. Vitamin C deficiency results in hemorrhage along with destructive and degenerative changes in the gingiva and underlying tissues and, as a result of this weakened tooth support, increased mobility. It does not, however, cause gingival inflammation. The initiation of gingival inflammation requires the presence of a local irritant. The inflammatory changes induced in the periodontal tissues by local irritating factors are different from those which result from acute vitamin C deficiency. In cases of periodontal disease in which both vitamin C deficiency and local irritating factors occur, the ability of the periodontal tissues to withstand the destructive effect of inflammation is impaired and the severity of the periodontal destruction is thereby increased.

There are specific histologic features that characterize the periodontal tissues in vitamin C deficiency and result in their lowered resistance to inflammation. These include a tendency toward collagen degeneration and failure to form new collagen, osteoporosis of alveolar bone, inability to produce well formed bone matrix and fewer blood vessels. When inflammation is superimposed upon vitamin C deficiency, the tissues have a reduced capacity to cope with this added problem as shown by their inability to form a peripheral delimitating connective tissue barrier to contain the inflammation. There is reduction in inflammatory cells, diminished vascular response and inhibition of both fibroblast formation and differentiation of cells to form osteoblasts.

Although vitamin C deficiency causes the connective tissue of the marginal gingiva to be altered by edema, collagen degeneration, and hemorrhage, the deficiency itself is not responsible for the initiation of, or an increase in, the incidence of marginal gingivitis. Periodontal pocket formation is not initiated by vitamin C deficiency. A complicating local factor is required before pocket formation occurs. However, when pocket formation does occur in vitamin C deficiency, it is of greater depth than that which usually occurs under comparable local conditions in the absence of this deficiency. This increased depth is related to the degenerative changes in the periodontal ligament which result from the vitamin C deficiency. By reducing the barrier formed by the dense collagen bundles normally found in this area, the migration of the epithelial attachment along the cementum is facilitated. The concomitant occurrence of both pocket formation and destruction of underlying tissues in vitamin C deficiency is not attributable to the deficiency alone but requires the presence of a complicating local factor.

Figure 104.   See illustrations on opposite page.

A. Control animal. Molar interdental bony septum showing well formed periodontal ligament fibers. Note osteoblasts along the mesial aspect of bone (left) and osteoclasts along the distal (right).

B. Vitamin C-deficient animal. Molar interdental bony septum showing edema and degeneration of periodontal ligament fibers. The bone margins are eroded throughout. The vessel channels are enlarged. There is no evidence of new bone formation.

C. Control animal. Incisor area, lingual aspect, showing division of periodontal ligament fibers into a vertical group (adjacent to tooth—left) and a horizontal group (adjacent to bone—right).

D. Vitamin C-deficient animal. Incisor area, lingual aspect, showing difference in the appearance of the periodontal ligament. Adjacent to the bone (right) there is hemorrhage and marked degeneration of the collagen. Adjacent to the tooth (left), the collagen presents comparatively slight degenerative change. Note eroded bone margin and break in the continuity of the collagen fibers and bone matrix.

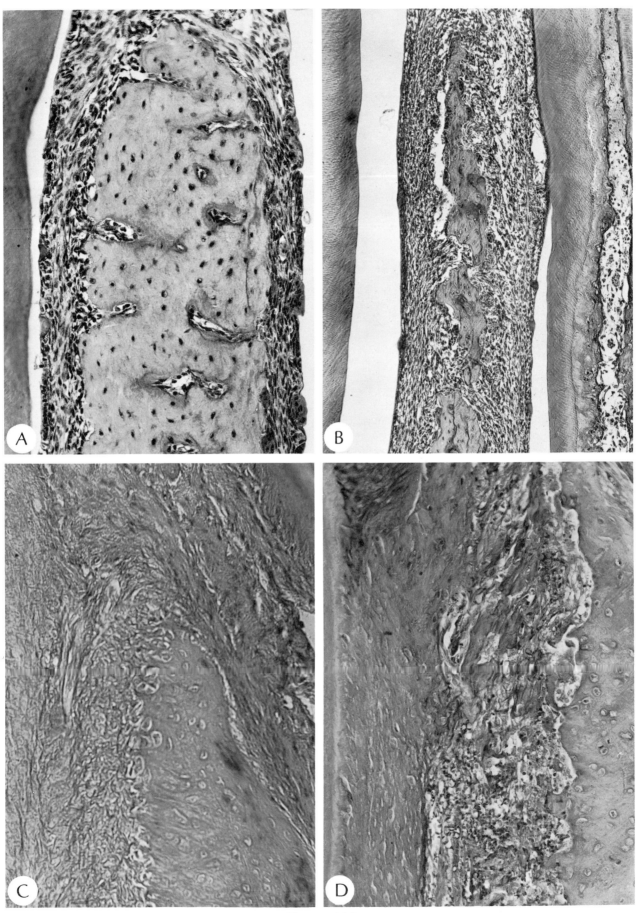

Figure 104

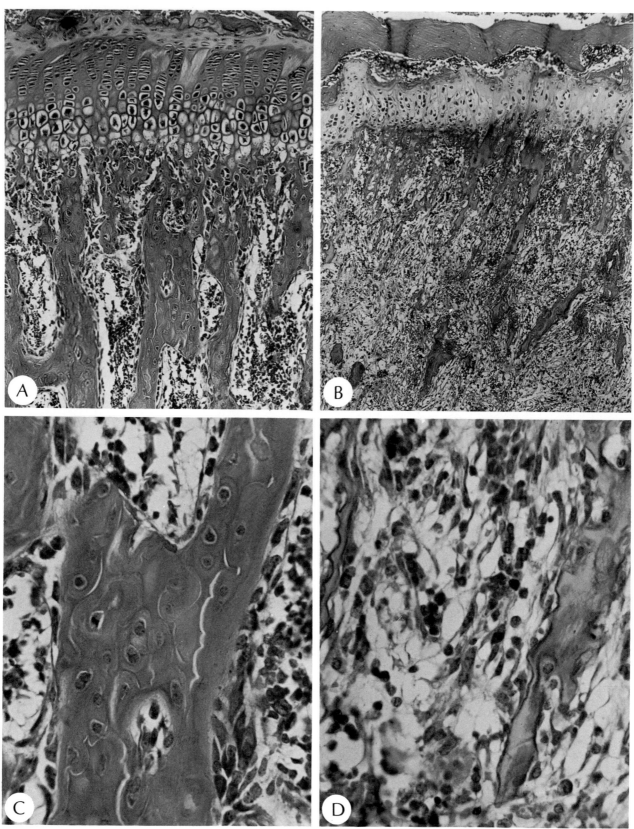

Figure 105

A. Control animal. Epidiaphyseal junction, distal end of femur showing regular arrangement of cartilage, cartilage cell changes, and contiguous bone trabeculae.

B. Vitamin C-deficient animal. Epidiaphyseal junction, distal end of femur showing irregular arrangement and distorted appearance of cartilage cells. Note thin bone trabeculae.

C. Control animal. Detail of A showing bone trabecula with adjacent osteoblasts and marginal osteoid matrix.

D. Vitamin C-deficient animal. Detail of B showing bone trabeculae with irregularly eroded margins and enlarged osteocyte lacunae. Note absence of osteoblasts and osteoid matrix.

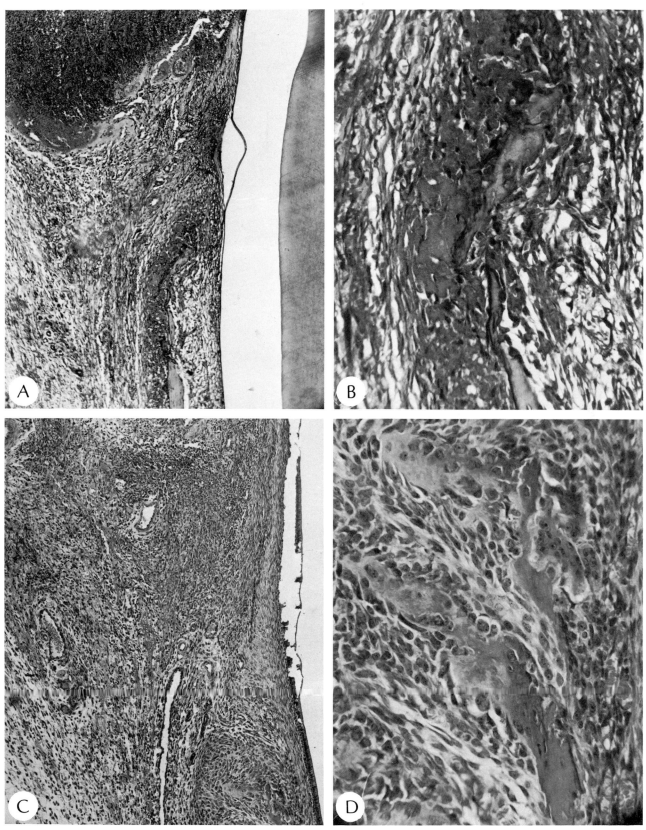

Figure 106

   A. Vitamin C-deficient animal. Labial surface of mandibular incisor showing area of necrosis at base of periodontal pocket and underlying connective tissue and bone.
   B. Vitamin C-deficient animal. Detail of A. Tip of alveolar plate showing degenerated collagen matrix adjoining osteoporotic alveolar bone. Note absence of osteoblasts and degeneration of surrounding periodontal ligament.
   C. Control animal. Area between base of periodontal pocket and underlying alveolar bone. Note concentration of inflammation beneath base of pocket.
   D. Control animal. Detail of C. Tip of labial plate showing alveolar bone, new bone formation, and osteoclasts. Note dense accumulation of connective tissue cells in areas of new bone formation.

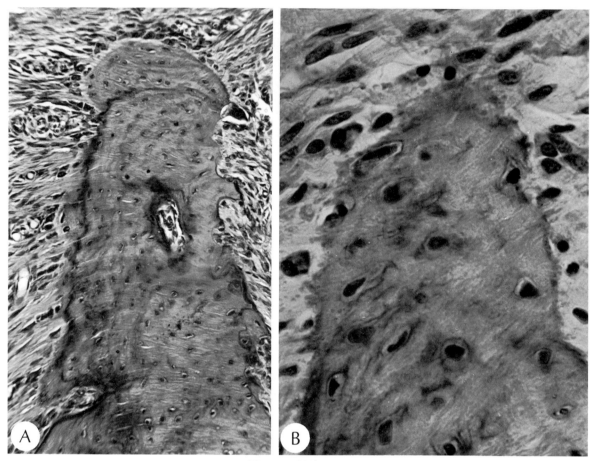

Figure 107

A. Control animal. Average blood sugar level 106 mg. per cent. Duration of experimental period: six weeks. Interdental septum of alveolar bone showing bone formation along mesial aspect (left). Resorption lacunae are seen along the distal aspect (right).

B. Diabetic animal. Average blood sugar level 260 mg. per cent. Crest of interdental septum showing fragmentation of bone matrix with release of osteocytes into surrounding connective tissue.

See illustrations on opposite page.

DIABETES

Chronic diabetes was induced in albino rats by injecting the drug alloxan. This resulted in a tendency toward generalized osteoporosis and a reduction in the height of the alveolar bone in 39 per cent of the animals. Comparable osteoporotic changes occurred in other bones of the skeletal system. Hyperglycemia and changes in the pancreas were not associated with a tendency toward osteoporosis in a specific cause and effect relationship. Chronic alloxan diabetes does not produce periodontal pockets nor changes in the periodontal ligament nor does it alter the incidence or severity of gingivitis.

Within limitations which govern the validity of correlations between the findings in animal experiments and disease as it occurs in humans, the following comments are offered regarding periodontal disease in human diabetes. In individual patients, diabetes is not responsible for specific gingival changes nor for the onset of gingivitis. Periodontitis in diabetic individuals presents no specific microscopic features which warrant its designation as a unique clinical entity. The existence of a basically unaltered condition throughout the alveolar bone in a large percentage of diabetics discourages the assumption that whenever periodontal disease occurs in diabetic individuals, its origin and progress are primarily generated by the diabetes. Control of the diabetes is an essential measure in the management of diabetic patients with periodontal disease but the elimination of the periodontitis is dependent upon removal of local factors.

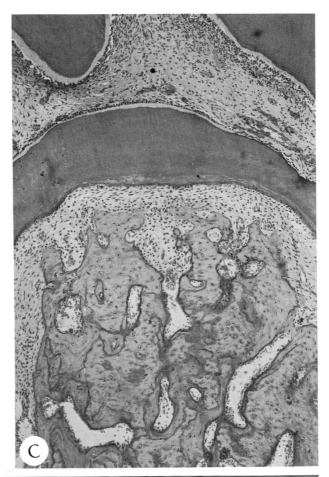

Legend continued.

   C. Diabetic animal. Average blood sugar level 260 mg. per cent. Duration of experimental period: eight weeks. Bifurcation area showing absence of bone formation adjacent to the periodontal ligament and along vessel channels and marrow spaces.

   D. Detail of C showing fragmentation of bone and release of osteocytes adjacent to the periodontal ligament. Some osteocytes are partially enclosed within a remnant of their lacunar wall and extend into the connective tissue.

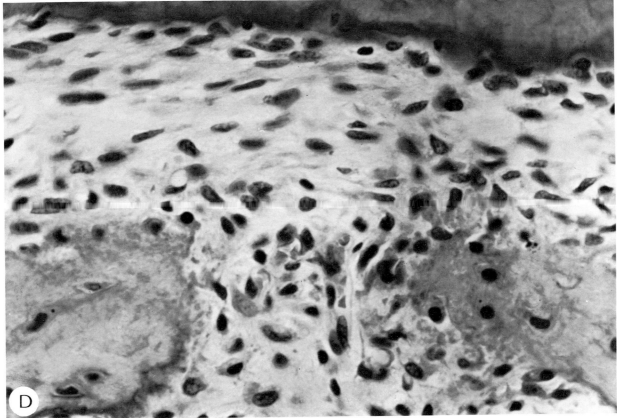

Figure 107

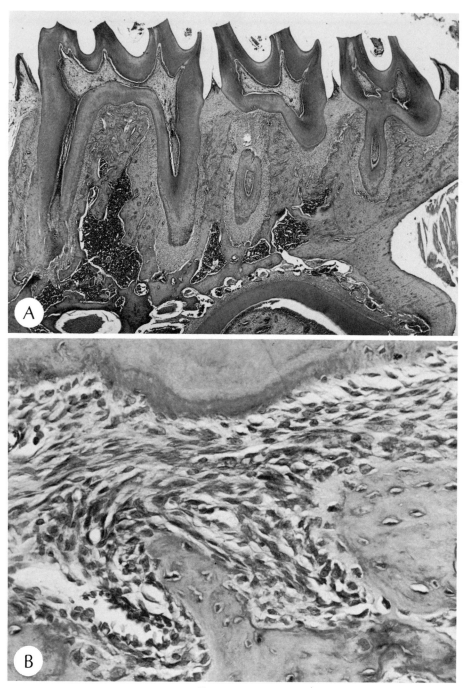

Figure 108

A. Control. Seven-day animal. Survey section of right mandibular molars.

B. Control. Seven-day animal. Crest of bone in first molar (left) bifurcation shown in A. Note cellularity of the periodontal ligament and adjacent bone and cementum formation.
See illustrations on opposite page.

DIABETES AND OCCLUSAL FORCES

An experiment was undertaken in rats that had been made diabetic to determine how the periodontal response to excessive occlusal forces would be affected by a systemic disturbance. Alloxan diabetes was selected because of its demonstrated effect upon the supporting periodontal tissues which is the area of the periodontium where trauma from occlusion is manifest.

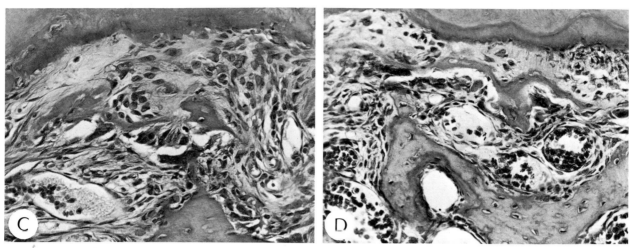

Figure 108

Legend continued.
    C. Occlusal trauma alone. Seven-day animal. Crest of bifurcation of mandibular first molar showing necrosis of the periodontal ligament and bone. There is fibroplasia and osteoblastic and osteoclastic activity.

    D. Alloxan plus occlusal trauma. Seven-day animal. Crest of bifurcation of mandibular first molar showing necrosis of the periodontal ligament and bone. There is only slight fibroplasia and osteoblastic activity. Compare with occlusal-trauma-alone animal (C).

    Alloxan diabetes aggravates and prolongs the effects of excessive occlusal forces by inhibiting repair of the lesions they produce. In all traumatized animals, both diabetic and non-diabetic, the injury occurred in the supporting periodontal tissues without unique gingival changes. The classical microscopic picture of trauma from occlusion was present. The periodontal ligament, bone and cementum in the bifurcation area is affected first as this area is most susceptible to injury from occlusal forces. By the seventh day, there is compression and necrosis of the periodontal ligament and adjacent bone, increased osteoblastic and osteoclastic activity, fibroplasia, reduction in the height of the crest and thickening of the periodontal ligament space, with resorption of cementum. Along the lateral aspect of the interradicular septa there is compression of the periodontal ligament. In non-diabetic animals the injury is repaired by the end of the second week, which is consistent with the reversibility of trauma from occlusion when the offending forces are dissipated. There is pronounced fibroplasia of the periodontal ligament and formation of trabeculae of new bone along the crest of the interradicular septum. The trabeculae are bordered by a well defined layer of osteoblasts and osteoid. New cementum fills the resorption lacunae and lines the cemental surface. In contrast to the non-diabetic animals, at the end of four months, the periodontium in the bifurcation of the traumatized diabetic animals is markedly different from the healed bifurcation in the non-diabetic traumatized animals. There is diminished fibroblastic activity in the periodontal ligament which impairs bone and cementum formation. The inability to re-create and sustain a well formed periodontal ligament results in a narrow periodontal space at the crest of the interradicular bone with some areas of contact between tooth and bone. With such defective support ordinary occlusal forces become injurious and an undesirable functional environment is perpetuated.

    Systemic influences affect the response of the periodontium to local environmental factors. The destructive effect of excessive occlusal forces upon the periodontium is aggravated in alloxan diabetes, protein deficient animals and by other abnormal metabolic states.

    Alloxan induced diabetes also affects the periodontal response to diminished occlusal function. It reduces osteoblastic and osteoclastic activity which ordinarily occurs around teeth of experimental animals with functionally extracted antagonists.

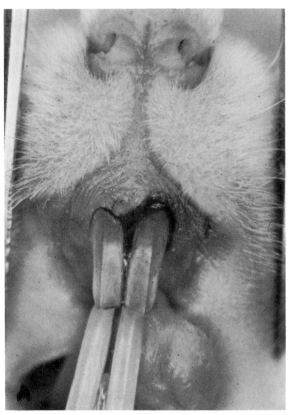

Figure 109

Rat immediately after surgical resection of marginal gingiva around maxillary left central incisor.

DIABETES AND PERIODONTAL HEALING

Diabetes retards healing following gingival surgery by inhibiting fibroblastic activity, collagen formation, the development of osteoblasts and new bone formation. It does not affect the epithelium nor the gingival sulcus. However, healing is influenced more by the direct effects of local irritants than the indirect effect of diabetes. Inflammation induced by local irritants retards healing by injuring the gingiva and underlying bone. Inflammation can also stimulate fibroplasia and bone formation, which overshadows the inhibitory effects of the diabetes upon the healing periodontium.

Figure 110.   See illustrations on opposite page.

A. Non-diabetic animal. Mandible seven days post-surgery. There is necrosis of the gingival margin and increased thickening of the labial bone.

B. Non-diabetic animal. Mandible seven days post-surgery. Detailed section of labial bone seen in A showing pronounced bone formative activity with new bone trabeculae extending labially from old bone.

C. Diabetic animal. Mandible seven days post-surgery. Dense suppurative inflammation replaces the marginal gingiva. The labial bone is necrotic at the crest, and thickened further apically along its labial aspect.

D. Diabetic animal. Mandible seven days post-surgery. Detailed view of C showing network of new trabeculae with pronounced osteoblastic activity on external surface of labial plate.

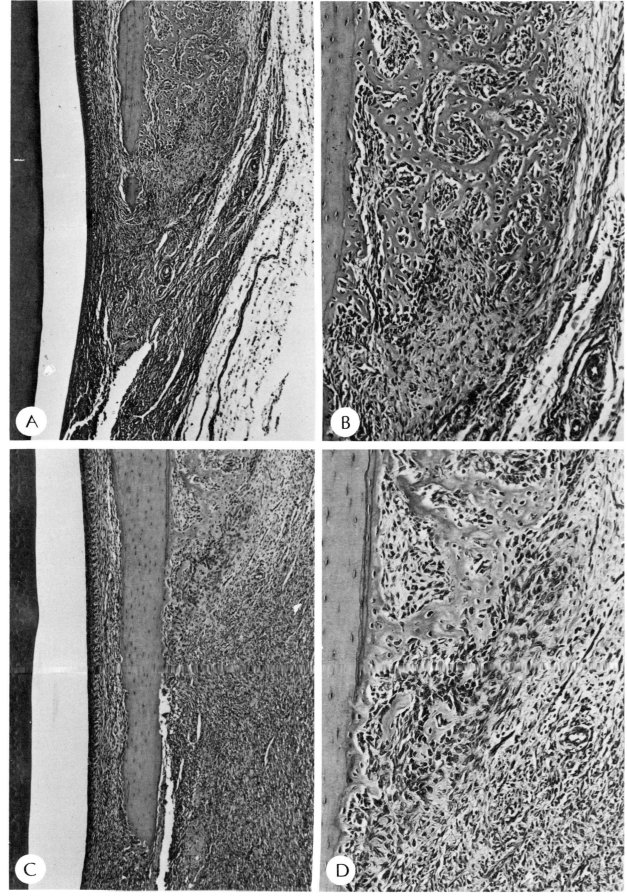

Figure 110

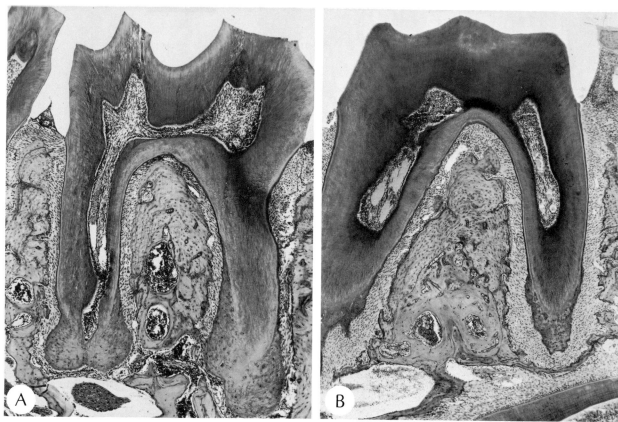

Figure 112

A. Control animal. Mesio-distal survey section through the mandibular first molar area.

B. Estrogen-injected animal. Mesio-distal survey section through the mandibular first molar area.

CORTISONE

In mice repeated daily injections of cortisone produce osteoporosis of the alveolar bone which is characterized by a reduction in the number of osteoblasts and amount of newly formed osteoid matrix. In addition, there is reduction in the height of the alveolar bone, edema of the periodontal ligament with reduction in the number of fibroblasts and degeneration of the collagen fibers. These changes take place unrelated to gingival inflammation which occurs in association with local irritation. Cortisone inhibits the fibroplasia which is necessary for the normal maintenance of the periodontal ligament and thereby produces the marked structural changes. The changes in the alveolar bone and periodontal ligament are comparable to those in the bone and periosteum in other areas of the skeletal system.

Figure 112.   See illustrations on opposite page.

C. Control animal. Detailed section of A showing the interradicular bone of the first molar. Three zones can be noted. In the mesial portion (right) note the spherical, irregularly arranged osteocytes and the irregularly indented margin in relation to the periodontal ligament. In the distal portion (left), note the coarsely fibrillar structure of the matrix and the osteocytes arranged in conformity with the incremental lines. In the central portion, note the concentric lamellations around the marrow spaces and the relative sparseness of cells as compared with the mesial and distal portions.

D. Estrogen-injected animal. Detailed section of B showing the interradicular bony septum. Note the sparse distribution of cells in the central portion and the clear demarcation of this area from the bone adjacent to the periodontal ligament. The absence of incremental or reversal lines in the central portion results in an appearance of uninterrupted homogeneity.

E. Cortisone-injected animal. Area comparable to that shown in C showing the interradicular bone of the first molar. Note the absence of bone formative activity along the endosteal margin of the marrow space.

F. Cortisone-estrogen animal. Area comparable to C showing the interradicular bone of the first molar. Note the irregular appearance of the recently formed bone bordering the marrow space.

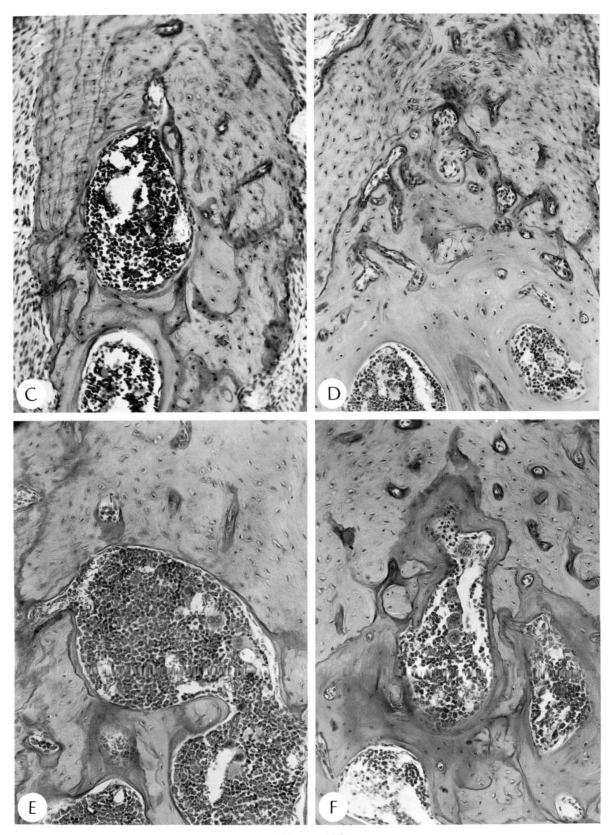

Figure 112

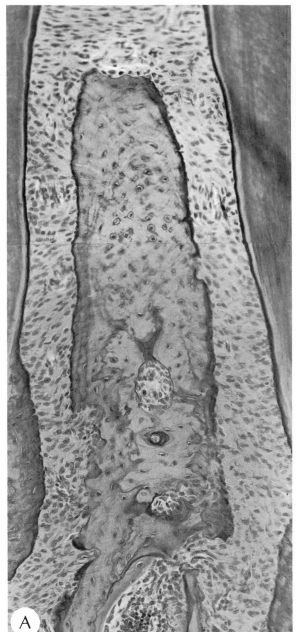

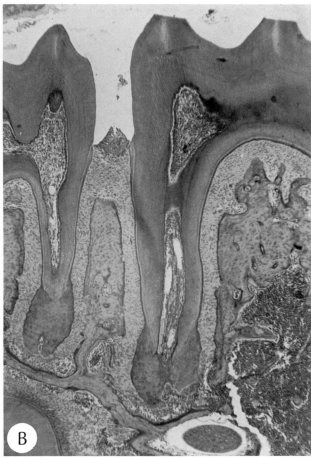

Figure 113

A. Cortisone-injected animal. Detailed section of B showing the interdental septum and periodontal ligament. The deeply staining distal (left) and mesial (right) surfaces of the interdental septum are devoid of any appreciable bone activity. The crest presents a flattened, indented margin. Note the peculiar grouping and sharply outlined ovoid lacunar spaces. Note, too, the irregularly indented margin of the medullary space in the central portion of the septum and the evidence of endosteal bone apposition bordering the medullary space in the lower region of the septum. With the exception of isolated areas, the periodontal ligament fibers are replaced by a homogeneous, minutely fibrillar stroma.

B. Cortisone-injected animal. Mesio-distal survey section through the mandible showing the interdental bone between the first and second molars.

See illustrations on opposite page.

CORTISONE MODIFIED BY ESTROGEN

Repeated injections with synthetic estrogen in male and female mice produce an initial increase in the cellularity of the periodontal ligament followed by a reduction in cellularity and collagen content and reduced alveolar bone formation. Endosteal bone formation is increased.

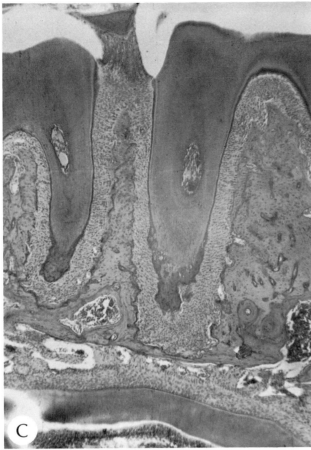

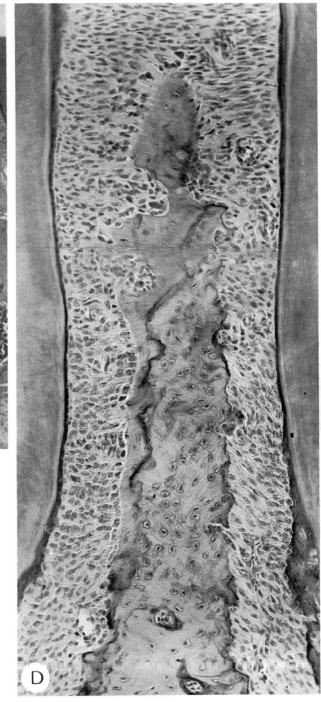

Figure 113

Legend continued.

    C. Cortisone-estrogen animal. Mesio-distal survey section through the mandible showing the interdental bone between the first and second molars.

    D. Cortisone-estrogen animal. Detailed section of C showing the interdental septum and periodontal ligament. Newly formed bone at the crest and along the distal surface (left) is demarcated from the underlying remainder of the septum by an irregular, deeply staining appositional line. Note the comparative abundance of osteocytes in the latter portion of the septum and the marked contrast between the mesial (right) and distal septal surfaces. The periodontal ligament contains numerous, large fibroblasts. The fibers are thin and strand-like in appearance. In some areas, it is difficult to note a demarcation of these strands into separate fibers or fiber bundles.

    Estrogen reverses the osteoporotic tendency induced by cortisone. Injecting estrogen in animals receiving cortisone results in renewed fibroplasia in the periodontal ligament, stimulation of bone formation and restoration in the height of previously reduced interdental bone.

    The periodontal ligament surfaces of the alveolar bone appear to be more sensitive to shifts in hormonal balance in either a positive or a negative direction than the remainder of the jaw because variations in occlusal function necessitate comparatively rapid adaptive changes in the distribution of bone along these surfaces.

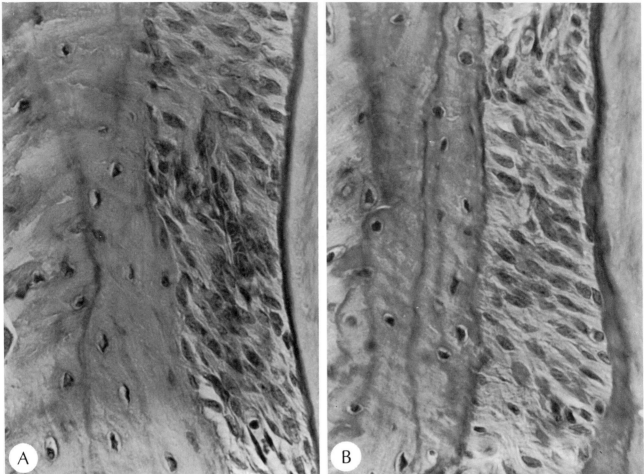

Figure 114

A. Control animal (five-week experimental period). Detailed section of distal surface of interdental septum, periodontal ligament and mesial surface of mesial root of the second mandibular molar. Note the smooth, regular outline of the alveolar bone with bordering osteoblasts.

B. Control animal (ten-week experimental period). Detailed section of distal surface of interdental septum and periodontal ligament between first and second mandibular molars in area comparable to that shown in A. Note the deeply staining linear borders of the alveolar bone and the reduction in osteoblasts (compare with A). The periodontal ligament presents well formed collagen and fibroblasts.

Figure 114. See illustrations on opposite page.

C. Estrogen-injected animal (five-week experimental period). Detailed section of distal surface on interdental septum and periodontal ligament between first and second mandibular molars in area comparable to that shown in A. The fibroblasts of the periodontal ligament appear to be increased in number. There is a layer of osteoid lined by a bead-like layer of osteoblasts along the border of the alveolar bone.

D. Estrogen-injected animal (ten-week experimental period). Detailed section of distal surface of interdental septum and periodontal ligament between first and second mandibular molars in area comparable to that shown in A. Note reduction in number of fibroblasts of the periodontal ligament and irregularly indented, darkly staining outline of the distal border of the alveolar septum. The collagen fibers appear reduced in amount, lightly staining, and fibrillar.

E. Cortisone-injected animal (five-week experimental period). Detailed section of distal surface of interdental septum and periodontal ligament between first and second molars in area comparable to that shown in A. Note reduction in number of fibroblasts of the periodontal ligament and irregularly indented, darkly staining outline of the distal border of the alveolar septum. The collagen fibers are reduced in amount. Note the relative absence of osteoblasts and new bone formation.

F. Cortisone-estrogen animal (five-week experimental period). Detailed section of distal surface of interdental septum and periodontal ligament between first and second mandibular molars in area comparable to that shown in A. Note newly formed bone along the surface of the septum and the prominent layer of osteoblasts.

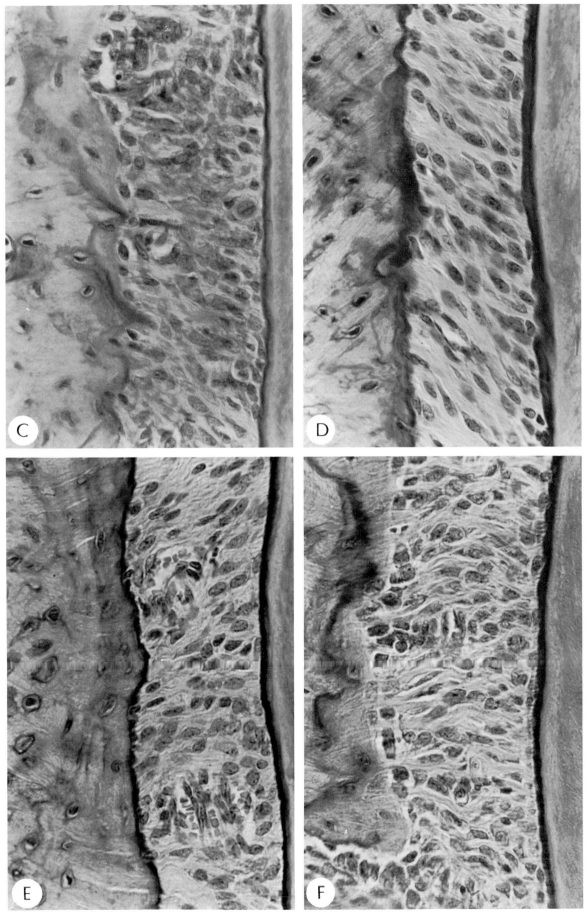

Figure 114

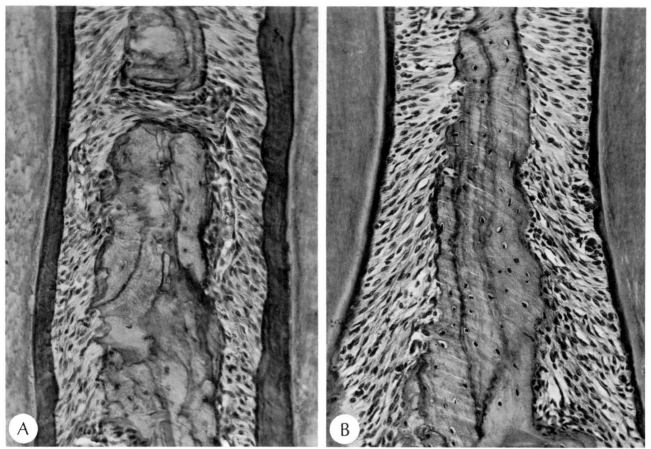

Figure 115

A. Control animal (four- to six-week group). Interdental septum between first (left) and second molars showing dense fibers in periodontal ligament, indented mesial margin of bone (left) and smooth distal margin with adjacent appositional lines.

B. Experimental animal (four- to six-week group). Interdental bone between first (left) and second molars. Note separation of periodontal ligament fibers, irregular distal margin of bone (right), and absence of appositional lines in distogingival area (top right).

OVARIECTOMY

Ovariectomy performed on young adult mice leads to osteoporotic changes in the alveolar bone and a reduction in density of the periodontal ligament fibers. When performed in animals at the age of physiologic cessation of the estrus, ovariectomy produces no changes in the alveolar bone. It would seem that the effect of ovariectomy on the bone in young animals is not a pathologic change, but rather a premature reduction in the anabolic activity to a level which is normal for older animals.

Figure 115.   See illustrations on opposite page.

C. Control animal (one-year group). Interdental septum between first (right) and second molars. Compare with B and note similarity.

D. Experimental animal (one-year group). Interdental septum between first (right) and second molars. There is no significant difference in this area between experimental and control animals. Compare with C.

E. Control animal (four- to six-week group). Crest of lingual alveolar plate, mandibular molar. Note normal distribution of osteoid and osteoblasts lining bone adjacent to the periodontal ligament.

F. Ovariectomized animal, six months after operation. Crest of lingual alveolar plate, mandibular molar. The bone formative activity normal for this area is absent. The periodontal ligament fibers are thinner, reduced in number and disorganized. The cellularity is diminished. Note the thin layer of cementum compared with control animal shown in E.

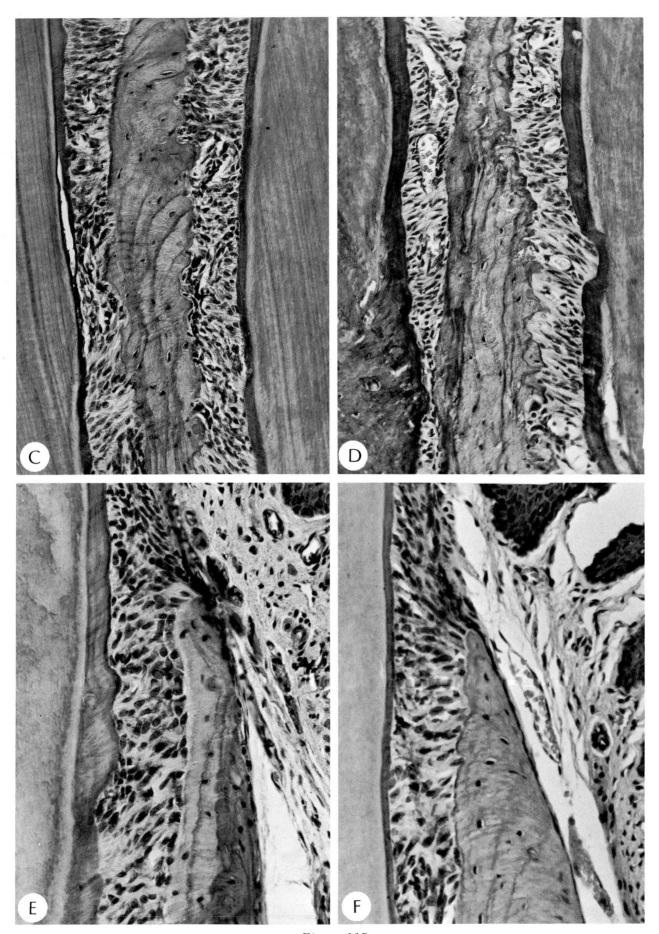

Figure 115

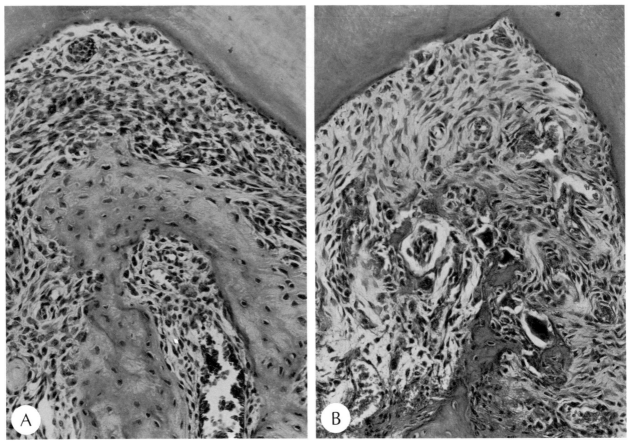

Figure 116

See legends on opposite page.

OSTEOLATHYRISM

Osteolathyrism is a skeletal disturbance induced experimentally in animals by feeding diets rich in *Lathyris odoratus* peas or by administering certain aminonitriles, such as aminoacetonitrile (AAN). It is used as a means to study bone changes. In osteolathyrism, the periosteum of the mandible is thickened and there are irregular bulbous exostoses along the lower and posterior borders in areas of muscle insertion. In some areas, the mandibular bone appears normal; in others, it is completely replaced by coarsely fibrillar bone with irregularly arranged trabeculae, lined with relatively acellular and deeply staining new bone.

The alveolar bone is osteoporotic with thinned irregular trabeculae and enlarged, engorged vessels. Osteoblasts and osteoclasts are increased in number adjacent to the periodontal ligament and along the endosteal margins. The osteoid matrix is increased in amount, deeply eosinophilic, and coarsely fibrillar.

The most severe changes occur in the furcation area. This is the region most sensitive to occlusal forces and there is general agreement that mechanical stress affects the location and severity of lathyritic changes.

In the gingiva there are fewer cells in the connective tissue and the collagen fibers are thinned and reduced in number. Inflammation is present but it is associated with local irritants.

In the periodontal ligament, the cellularity and fiber content are decreased and the fiber bundle arrangement is partially disorganized. There are areas in which the fibers are extremely dense with patchy areas of hyalinization, bordered by palisading connective tissue cells. The transseptal fibers are thinned and hyalinized at the area of insertion into the cementum.

In the cementum there are numerous areas of resorption that often extend into the dentin. Cementum apposition at the apices is retarded and abnormal. Cementoblasts are reduced in number and irregularly aligned on the root surface. The deeply staining eosinophilic precementum is fibrillar and irregularly distributed. In the formed cementum, the cells are reduced in number and irregular in distribution.

Lathyritic changes can be aggravated by systemic disturbances such as partial hepatectomies and thyroparathyroidectomies and ameliorated by the administration of thyroxin and ACTH.

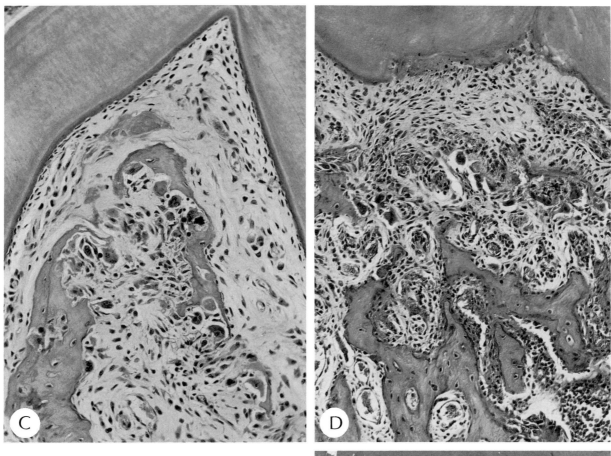

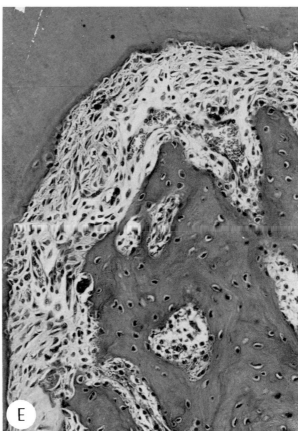

A. Untreated control. Bifurcation area of first molar showing normal periodontal ligament and bone formation.

B. AAN-treated. Bifurcation area of first molar showing altered periodontal ligament, widened periodontal ligament space, abnormal osteoid formation, osteoclasis and resorption of cementum and dentin.

C. AAN plus thyroparathyroidectomy plus 1 μg. thyroxin/day. Bifurcation of first molar showing pronounced hyalinization of the periodontal ligament, reduced cellularity, and marked osteoporosis.

D. AAN plus partial hepatectomies. Bifurcation of first molar showing hyalinization of the periodontal ligament, reduction in cellularity, pronounced osteoporosis, and abnormal osteoid.

E. AAN plus thyroxin 500 μg./day. Bifurcation of first molar showing slight lathyritic changes such as hyalinization of the periodontal ligament and abnormal osteoid. Compare with B, C and D.

Figure 116

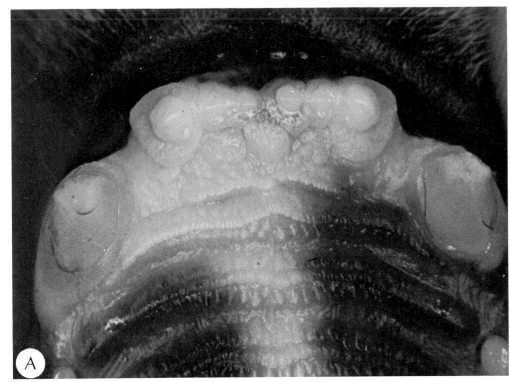

Figure 118

A. Experimental animal 166 days after administration of Dilantin. Palatal view showing pronounced gingival enlargement with minutely lobulated surface.

See illustrations on opposite page.

DILANTIN HYPERPLASIA

Hyperplasia of the gingiva is one of the side effects that may occur from the use of Dilantin (diphenylhydantoin sodium), a drug that is frequently used in the treatment of epilepsy. It is important, therefore, to understand the histological changes involved in the initiation and enlargement of the gingiva, the region of the periodontium in which the lesion originates and its relationship to local irritation. Since cats are susceptible to Dilantin-induced gingival hyperplasia, they provide a useful experimental model for the study of this problem.

Enlargement begins in some Dilantin-fed animals with only the slightest microscopic evidence of inflammation but does not occur in others with pronounced grossly visible gingival inflammation. Inflammation is a complication of gingival enlargement associated with Dilantin rather than an initiating factor. The gingival enlargement associated with Dilantin is a marginal proliferative lesion. It affects only the marginal and interproximal gingiva, without appreciable extension into the adjacent attached gingiva, underlying periodontal tissues and remainder of the oral mucosa. The gross appearance of the gingiva reflects the microscopic changes in the various stages. Initially, the interproximal and marginal gingiva are slightly enlarged, containing engorged prominent capillaries and numerous proliferating fibroblasts in a meshwork of collagen strands. In the second stage, red bead-like masses appear as protrusions from under the gingival margin. A slight linear depression demarcates the protruding masses from the gingival margin. In the final stage, the enlarged gingiva extends labially, lingually and interproximally, partially obscuring the teeth from view. It is composed of densely collagenous tissue covered by hyperplastic stratified squamous epithelium. When uncomplicated by inflammation the enlarged gingiva is pink and firm. The color and consistency change in the presence of accumulated local irritants.

The mechanism whereby gingival enlargement is produced by Dilantin is not understood. The peculiar susceptibility of the marginal and interproximal gingiva, the absence of changes in the remainder of the oral mucosa, the disappearance of the lesion after the teeth are extracted, and the immunity of some individuals to Dilantin-induced gingival enlargement are provocative aspects of the problem.

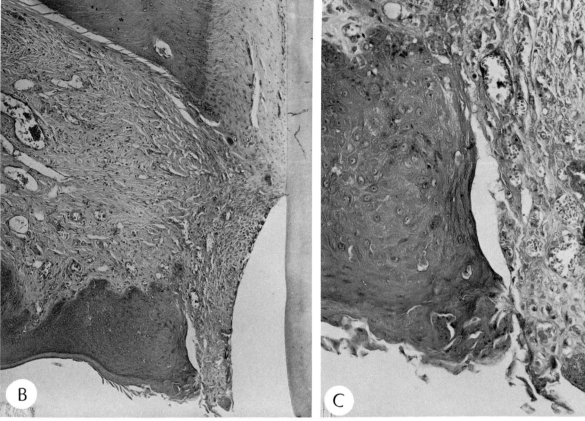

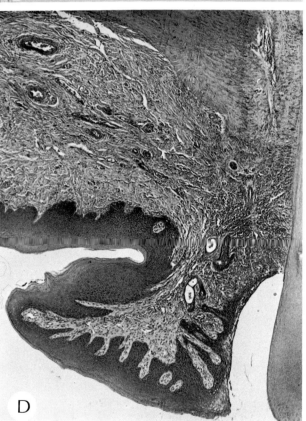

Legend continued.

B. Experimental animal 5 days after the administration of Dilantin. Labio-palatal section of palatal marginal gingiva of the maxillary right third incisor. The gingiva is wedged aside and the connective tissue has protruded beyond the margin.

C. Experimental animal 5 days after the administration of Dilantin. Detailed view of palatal gingival margin shown in B. Note the proliferating fibroblasts, collagen and capillaries. Remnants of degenerated epithelial cells are seen along the inner surface of the connective tissue facing the tooth surface. The gingival epithelium adjacent to this extruding mass is clearly demarcated from it and acanthotic.

D. Experimental animal 166 days after administration of Dilantin. Labio-palatal section of the maxillary right third incisor with bulbous marginal enlargement of the gingiva. Leukocytic infiltration is concentrated at the base of the sulcus. Note hyperplastic epithelium.

Figure 118

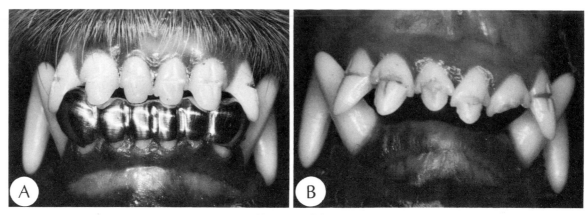

Figure 124

A. Cast overcontoured splint in dog to create hyperfunction. Notches in teeth are for clinical measurements.

B. Hypofunction in dog created by extraction of mandibular anterior teeth. Notches in teeth are for clinical measurements.

See illustrations on opposite page.

MUCOGINGIVAL SURGERY AND OCCLUSAL FORCES

Severe abnormal occlusal conditions significantly affect healing following mucogingival surgery operations in which the periosteum is removed from the bone and in which the periosteum is left intact. The effects are manifested in the periodontal ligament and alveolar bone. Changes in occlusal forces apparently do not influence the healing of the gingiva in terms of the formation of a normal gingival sulcus, zone of attached gingiva and location of the gingival attachment on the root surface.

In animals with reduced function there is reorientation in direction of the periodontal ligament fibers and a reduction in fiber density. The alveolar crest fibers are longer than normal and extend from the crest of the alveolar bone to the tooth surface almost parallel to it, which is consistent with extrusion of the tooth.

In animals with excess function, the periodontal ligament is densely fibrous, widened, and more vascular. The bone surface adjacent to the periodontal ligament is remodeled as evidenced by new bone and osteoid in previously resorbed areas. On the palatal surface of the teeth in hyperfunction there are well formed periodontal ligament fibers with new bone increments suggesting a response to tension created by excessive labially directed forces.

The most striking change created by the abnormal occlusion is the altered contour of the labial plate in the operated areas. Comparable changes in contour occur with reduced and excess function and with both periosteum removed and retained operations. The changes consist of a thinning and a tapering of the gingival segment of the labial plate and a bulge-like thickening in the apical portion. The thinning of the bone results from increased osteoclasis along the outer surface, and the thickening is produced by periosteal bone apposition.

It appears that the altered occlusion does not cause reduction in bone height beyond that produced by the experimental surgical procedures. In all operated animals the labial bone height was reduced to a greater degree with the repositioned flap, periosteum removed from the bone operation than with the resected gingival flap, periosteum intact on the bone operation.

Extreme and abrupt alterations in occlusion affect healing and bone contour following mucogingival surgery and the effects are microscopically detectable three months after operation. Less severe and gradual changes in occlusal forces might be tolerated without affecting postsurgical healing. Occlusal forces constitute a variable which can affect healing following mucogingival surgery.

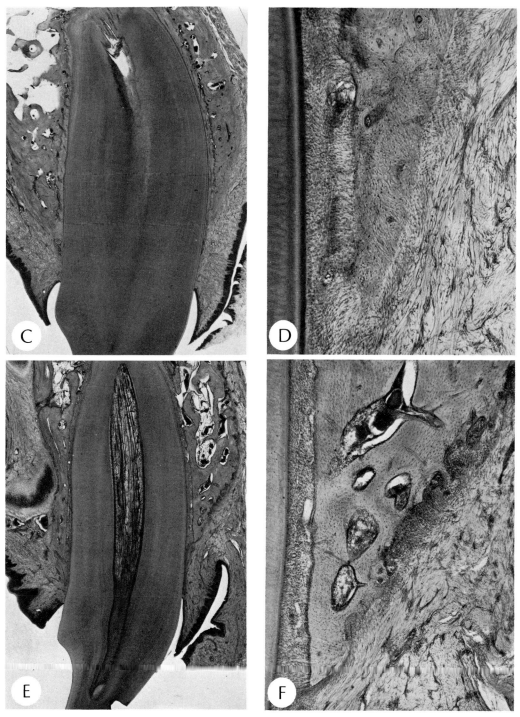

Figure 124

Legend continued.

    C. Unaltered occlusion – Resected gingival flap operation – Periosteum intact on the bone. Survey labio-palatal section of right maxillary incisor three months after operation showing increased length of attached gingiva and slight reduction in height of labial bone.

    D. Unaltered occlusion. Detailed view of labial crest shown in C. Note dense periodontal ligament fiber bundles perpendicular to tooth and bone with bone formation adjacent to periodontal ligament and on external labial surface.

    E. Hypofunction animal. Resected gingival flap operation – Periosteum intact on the bone. Survey labio-palatal section of right maxillary incisor three months after operation. There is slight reduction in height of labial bone with thinning of the gingival portion and thickening in the apical half.

    F. Hypofunction animal. Detailed view of crest of labial bone shown in E. There is a reduction in the number and density of the periodontal ligament fibers. Note resorption of bone on external surface.

References

GINGIVAL AND PERIODONTAL
DISEASE—INTRODUCTION (See page 1.)

Glickman, I.: Periodontal disease. N. Engl. J. Med., 284:1071, 1971.

United States Department of Health, Education, and Welfare. Public Health Service: Research Explores Pyorrhea and Other Gum Diseases: Periodontal Disease. Washington, D.C. Government Printing Office, 1970 (PHS Publication No. 1482).

United States National Center for Health Statistics. Vital and Health Statistics. Kelly, J. E., and Van Kirk, L. E.: Periodontal Disease in Adults: United States—1960-1962. Washington, D.C. Government Printing Office, 1965 (PHS Publication No. 1000, Series 11, No. 12).

Scherp, H. W.: Current concepts in periodontal disease research: Epidemiological contributions. J. Am. Dent. Assoc., 68:667, 1964.

Allen, E. F.: Statistical study of the primary causes of extractions. J. Dent. Res., 23:453, 1944.

Goldman, H. M.: Prevalence of parodontal (periodontal) disease. 4. In the United States. Int. Dent. J., 5:458, 1955.

Russell, A. L.: Epidemiology of periodontal disease. Int. Dent. J., 17:282, 1967.

Pelton, W. J., Pennell, E. H., and Druzina, A.: Tooth morbidity experience in adults. J. Am. Dent. Assoc., 49:439, 1954.

NORMAL GINGIVA—CLINICAL (See pages 2 and 3.)

Ainamo, J., and Löe, H.: Anatomical characteristics of gingiva. A clinical and microscopic study of the free and attached gingiva. J. Periodontol., 37:5, 1966.

Cabrini, R. L., and Carranza, F. A., Jr.: Histochemistry of periodontal tissues. A review of the literature. Int. Dent. J., 16:466, 1966.

Forsslund, G.: Structure and function of the capillary system in the gingiva in man. Development of a stereophotogrammetric method and its application for study of the subepithelial blood vessels in vivo. Acta Odontol. Scand., 17:9, Suppl. 26, 1960.

Fullmer, H. M.: A critique of normal connective tissue of the periodontium and some alterations with periodontal disease. J. Dent Res., 41:223, 1962.

Greene, A. H.: A study of the characteristics of stippling and its relation to gingival health. J. Periodontol., 33:176, 1962.

Kindlova, M.: The blood supply of the marginal periodontium in macacus rhesus. Arch. Oral. Biol., 10:869, 1965.

Rosenberg, H., and Massler, M.: Gingival stippling in young adult males. J. Periodontol., 38:473, 1967.

GINGIVAL PIGMENTATION (See page 4.)

Bolden, T. E.: Histology of oral pigmentation. J. Periodontol., 31:361, 1960.

Dummett, C. O.: Oral pigmentation. J. Periodontol., 31:356, 1960.

GINGIVA—HISTOCHEMICAL STAINS (See page 5.)

Orban, B.: Clinical and histologic study of the surface characteristics of the gingiva. Oral Surg., 1:827, 1948.

Owings, J. R.: A clinical investigation of the relationship between stippling and surface keratinization of the attached gingiva. J. Periodont.-Periodontics, 40:588, 1969.

GINGIVA—HISTOLOGY (See pages 6 and 7.)

Turesky, S., Glickman, I., and Litwin, T.: A histochemical evaluation of normal and inflamed human gingiva. J. Dent. Res., 30:792, 1951.

GINGIVAL FIBERS (See pages 8 and 9.)

Goldman, H.: The topography and role of the gingival fibers. J. Dent. Res., 30:331, 1951.

Arnim, S. S., and Hagerman, D. A.: The connective tissue fibers of the marginal gingiva. J. Am. Dent. Assoc., 47:271, 1953.

GINGIVAL SULCUS (See pages 10 and 11.)

Gottlieb, B.: Epithelansatz am Zahne. Deutsch. Monatschr. f. Zahnhk., 39:142, 1921.

Weski, O.: Die chronischen marginalen entzundungen

des alveolar-fort satzes mit besonderer beruck-sichtigung der Alveolar pyorrhoe. Vertelahrschr. f. Zahnheilk., 38:1, 1922.

Waerhaug, J.: Current views on the epithelial cuff. Periodontics, 4:278, 1966.

Listgarten, M. A.: Changing concepts about the dento-epithelial junction. J. Can. Dent. Assoc., 36:70, 1970.

Engler, W. O., Ramfjord, S. P., and Hiniker, J. J.: Development of epithelial attachment and gingival sulcus in rhesus monkeys. J. Periodontol., 34:44, 1965.

Engler, W. O., Ramfjord, S. P., and Hiniker, J. J.: Healing following simple gingivectomy. A tritiated thymidine autoradiographic study. I. Epithelialization. J. Periodontol., 37:298, 1966.

Cran, J. A.: Development of the gingival sulcus. Aust. Dent. J., 11:322, 1966.

Löe, H., and Holm-Pedersen, P.: Absence and presence of fluid from normal and inflamed gingivae. Periodontics, 3:171, 1965.

Björn, A. L., Koch, G., and Lindhe, J.: Evaluation of gingival fluid measurements. Odontol. Rev., 16:300, 1965.

Brandtzaeg, P.: Pocket fluid, serum and saliva. Arch. Oral Biol., 10:795, 1965.

CUTICLES (See pages 12 and 13.)

Listgarten, M. A.: Changing concepts about the dento-epithelial junction. J. Can. Dent. Assoc., 36:70, 1970.

Listgarten, M. A.: Phase contrast and electron microscopic study of the junction between reduced enamel epithelium and enamel in unerupted human teeth. Arch. Oral Biol., 11:999, 1966.

Wertheimer, F. W.: A histologic comparison of apical cuticles, secondary dental cuticles and hyaline bodies. J. Periodontol., 37:91, 1966.

Wertheimer, F. W., and Fullmer, H. M.: Morphologic and histochemical observations on the human dental cuticle. J. Periodontol., 33:29, 1962.

ELECTRON MICROSCOPY — NORMAL AND INFLAMED GINGIVA (See pages 14–21.)

Susi, F.: Histochemical, autoradiographic and electron microscopic studies of keratinization in oral mucosa. Ph.D. Thesis, Tufts University, October, 1967.

Stern, I. B.: Electron microscopic observations of oral epithelium. I. Basal cells and the basement membrane. Periodontics, 3:224, 1965.

Schroeder, H. E., and Listgarten, M. A.: Fine structure of the developing epithelial attachment of human teeth. (Monographs in developmental biology, Vol. 2.) Basel, New York, Karger, 1971.

PLAQUE — PELLICLE — MATERIA ALBA (See pages 22 and 23.)

Gibbons, R. L.: Dental Plaque. Edited by W. D. McHugh. London. E. & S. Livingstone Co., 1970.

Jenkins, G. N.: The chemistry of plaque. Ann. NY Acad. Sci., 131:786, 1965.

Löe, H., Theilade, E., and Jensen, S. B.: Experimental gingivitis in man. J. Periodontol., 37:177, 1965.

Mandel, I. D.: Dental plaque: Nature, formation and effects. J. Periodontol., 37:357, 1966.

Mandel, I. D.: Plaque and calculus measurements — Rate of formation and pathogenic potential. J. Periodontol., 38:721, 1967.

Turesky, S., Gilmore, N. D., and Glickman, I.: Reduced plaque formation by the chloromethyl analogue of Victamine C. J. Periodontol., 41:41, 1970.

CALCULUS (See pages 24 and 25.)

Conroy, C., and Sturzenberger, O.: The rate of calculus formation in adults. J. Periodontol., 39:142, 1968.

Everett, F. G., Tuchler, H., and Lu, K. H.: Occurrence of calculus in grade school children in Portland, Oregon. J. Periodontol., 34:54, 1963.

Kopczyk, R., and Conroy, C.: The attachment of calculus to root planed surfaces. Periodontics, 6:78, 1968.

Leung, S. W.: Naturally occurring stains on the teeth of children. J. Am. Dent. Assoc., 41:191, 1950.

Schroeder, H. E.: Formation and inhibition of dental calculus. Bern, Huber, 1969.

Turesky, S., Renstrup, G., and Glickman, I.: Effects of changing the salivary environment upon the progress of calculus formation. J. Periodontol., 33:45, 1962.

INTERDENTAL (COL) AREA (See pages 26–30.)

Cohen, B.: Morphological factors in the pathogenesis of periodontal disease. Br. Dent. J., 107:31, 1959.

Fish, W.: Etiology and prevention of periodontal breakdown. Dent. Prog., 1:234, 1961.

McHugh, W. D.: The development of the gingival epithelium in the monkey. Dent. Pract., Dent. Rec., 11:314, 1961.

Stahl, S. S.: Morphology and healing pattern of human interdental gingivae. J. Am. Dent. Assoc., 67:48, 1963.

Melcher, A. H.: Lesions of the interdental gingival septum and their effect on therapeutic procedures. A preliminary report. J. Periodontol., 33:311, 1962.

GINGIVA — INFLAMMATORY CELLS (See pages 32–34.)

Melcher, A. H.: Some histological and histochemical observations on the connective tissue of chronically inflamed human gingiva. J. Periodont. Res., 2:127, 1967.

Zachrisson, B. U.: Mast cells of the human gingiva. 2. Metachromatic cells at low pH in healthy and inflamed tissue. J. Periodont. Res., 2:87, 1967.

Zachrisson, B. U., and Schultz-Haudt, S. D.: A comparative histological study of clinically normal and chronically inflamed gingivae from the same individuals. Odont. T., 76:179, 1968.

Dewar, M. R.: Observations on the composition and

metabolism of normal and inflamed gingivae. J. Periodontol., 26:29, 1955.

INTERDENTAL PAPILLA — INFLAMMATION (See pages 34–37.)

Holmes, C. H.: Morphology of the interdental papillae. J. Periodontol., 36:455, 1965.

Kohl, J. T., and Zander, H. A.: Morphology of the interdental gingival tissues. Oral Surg., 14:287, 1961.

McHugh, W. D.: The interdental gingivae. J. Periodont. Res., 6:227, 1971.

World Workshop in Periodontics, Edited by Ramfjord, S. P., Kerr, A., and Ash, M. M., Ann Arbor, Michigan, University of Michigan, 1966, p. 171.

Stahl, S. S.: Morphology and healing pattern of human interdental gingivae. J. Am. Dent. Assoc., 67:48, 1963.

Levin, M. A.: The interdental papillae in gingivitis — A review survey. J. Periodontol., 37:230, 1966.

GINGIVA — CHILDREN (See pages 38 and 39.)

Zappler, S. E.: Periodontal disease in children. J. Am. Dent. Assoc., 37:333, 1948.

Gupta, O. P.: An epidemiological study of periodontal disease in Trivandrum, India. J. Dent. Res., 43:876, 1964.

Bradley, R. E.: Periodontal lesions of children: Their recognition and treatment. Dent. Clin. North Am., November, 1961, p. 671.

Massler, M., Cohen, A., and Schour, I.: Epidemiology of gingivitis in children. J. Am. Dent. Assoc., 45:319, 1952.

GINGIVITIS — EARLY (See page 40.)

Hoover, D. R., and Lefkowitz, W.: Fluctuation in marginal gingivitis. J. Periodontol., 36:310, 1965.

Larato, D. C., Stahl, S. S., Brown, R., Jr., and Witkin, G. J.: The effect of a prescribed method of toothbrushing on the fluctuation of marginal gingivitis. J. Periodont.-Periodontics, 40:142, 1969.

Hock, J., and Niki, K.: A vital microscopy study of the morphology of normal and inflamed gingiva. J. Periodont. Res., 6:81, 1971.

GINGIVITIS — RECESSION (See pages 41–43.)

Gorman, W. J.: Prevalence and etiology of gingival recession. J. Periodontol., 38:316, 1967.

Kitchen, P. C.: The prevalence of tooth root exposure and the relation of the extent of such exposure to the degree of abrasion in different age classes. J. Dent. Res., 20:565, 1941.

Gottlieb, B., and Orban, B.: Active and passive continuous eruptions of the teeth. J. Dent. Res., 13:214, 1933.

Bass, C. C.: A demonstrable line on extracted teeth indicating the location of the outer border of the epithelial attachment. J. Dent. Res., 25:401, 1946.

Stillman, P. R., and McCall, J. O.: A Textbook of Clinical Periodontia. 2nd Edition, New York, MacMillan, 1937.

GINGIVAL ENLARGEMENT (See pages 44–47.)

Emslie, R. E., Massler, M., and Zwemer, J. D.: Mouth breathing: I. Etiology and effects. J. Am. Dent. Assoc., 44:506, 1952.

Glickman, I.: A basic classification of gingival enlargement. J. Periodontol., 21:131, 1950.

Glickman, I.: Clinical Periodontology, 4th Edition, Philadelphia, W. B. Saunders, 1972.

Ramfjord, S. P.: The histopathology of inflammatory gingival enlargement. Oral Surg., 6:516, 1953.

DILANTIN HYPERPLASIA (See pages 48 and 49.)

Babcock, J. R.: Incidence of gingival hyperplasia associated with Dilantin therapy in a hospital population. J. Am. Dent. Assoc., 71:1447, 1965.

Glickman, I., and Lewitus, M.: Hyperplasia of the gingivae associated with Dilantin (sodium diphenyl hydantoinate) therapy. J. Am. Dent. Assoc., 28:199, 1941.

Panuska, H. J., Gorlin, R. J., Bearman, J. E., and Mitchell, D. F.: The effect of anti-convulsant drugs upon the gingiva — A series of 1048 patients. II. J. Periodontol., 32:15, 1961.

BLOOD DYSCRASIAS (See pages 50 and 51.)

Burket, L. W.: A histopathologic explanation for the oral lesions in the acute leukemias. Am. J. Orthodont. & Oral Surg., 30:516, 1944.

Beck, L.: Thrombocytopenic purpura. Oral Surg., 15:148, 1962.

Anday, G. J.: Blood dyscrasias and their relationship to the dentist. J. Am. Dent. Assoc., 31:1458, 1944.

Lynch, M. A., and Ship, I.: Initial oral manifestations of leukemia. J. Am. Dent. Assoc., 75:932, 1967.

Lynch, M. A., and Ship, I.: Oral manifestations of leukemia: A postdiagnostic study. J. Am. Dent. Assoc., 75:1139, 1967.

HORMONAL CHANGES (See pages 52 and 53.)

Cohen, M. M.: The gingiva at puberty. J. Dent. Res., 34:679, 1955.

Cohen, D. W., Friedman, L., Shapiro, J., and Kyle, G. C.: A longitudinal investigation of the periodontal changes during pregnancy. J. Periodont.-Periodontics, 40:563, 1969.

Löe, H.: Periodontal changes in pregnancy. J. Periodontol., 36:209, 1965.

Ziskin, D. E., and Nesse, G. J.: Pregnancy gingivitis: history, classification, etiology. Am. J. Orthodont. & Oral Surg., 32:390, 1946.

ORAL SURGERY

Hugoson, A.: Gingival inflammation and female sex hormones. J. Periodont. Res., Suppl. 5:1, 1970.

ACUTE NECROTIZING ULCERATIVE GINGIVITIS (See pages 54–56.)

Goldhaber, P., and Giddon, D. B.: Present concepts concerning the etiology and treatment of acute necrotizing ulcerative gingivitis. Int. Dent. J., *14*:468, 1964.

Formicola, A. J., Witte, E. T., and Curran, P. M.: A study of personality traits and acute necrotizing ulcerative gingivitis. J. Periodontol., *41*:36, 1970.

King, J. D.: Nutritional and other factors in "trench mouth," with special reference to the nicotinic acid component of vitamin B₂ complex. Br. Dent. J., *74*:113, 1943.

Listgarten, M. A., and Lewis, D. W.: The distribution of spirochetes in the lesion of acute necrotizing ulcerative gingivitis: An electron microscopic and statistical survey. J. Periodontol., 38:379, 1967.

Rosebury, T.: Is Vincent's infection a communicable disease? J. Am. Dent. Assoc., 29:823, 1942.

Škach, M., Zábrodsky, S., and Mrklas, L.: A study of the effect of age and season on the incidence of ulcerative gingivitis. J. Periodont. Res., 5:187, 1970.

PERICORONITIS (See pages 57–59.)

Ash, M. M.: Third molars as periodontal problems. Dent. Clin. North Am., March, 1964, p. 51.

Braden, B. E.: Deep distal pockets adjacent to terminal teeth. Dent. Clin. North Am., *13*:161, 1969.

Blair, V. P.: The gingival operculum and the erupting lower third molar. Arch. Clin. Oral Path., *4*:283, 1940.

ABSCESS (See pages 60–63.)

Trott, J. R.: Acute periodontal abscess. J. Can. Dent. Assoc., 25:601, 1959.

DESQUAMATIVE GINGIVITIS (See pages 64–66.)

Brusati, R., and Bracchetti, A.: Electron microscopic study of chronic desquamative gingivitis. J. Periodont.-Periodontics, *40*:388, 1969.

Engel, M., Ray, H. G., and Orban, B.: The pathogenesis of desquamative gingivitis. A disturbance of the connective tissue ground substance. J. Dent. Res., 29:410, 1950.

Glickman, I., and Smulow, J. B.: Histopathology and histochemistry of chronic desquamative gingivitis. Oral Surg., *21*:325, 1966.

McCarthy, F. P., McCarthy, P. L., and Shklar, G.: Chronic desquamative gingivitis: A reconsideration. Oral Surg., *13*:1300, 1960.

Glickman, I., and Smulow, J. B.: Chronic desquamative gingivitis—Its nature and treatment. J. Periodontol., *35*:397, 1964.

LEUKOPLAKIA – HYPERKERATOSIS (See pages 68 and 69.)

Darling, A. I., and Fletcher, J. P.: Familial white folded gingivostomatitis. Oral Surg., *11*:296, 1958.

Renstrup, G.: Leukoplakia of the oral cavity. A clinical and histopathologic study. Acta Odontol. Scand., *16*:99, 1958.

Silverman, S., Jr., and Rozen, R. D.: Observations on the clinical characteristics and natural history of oral leukoplakia. J. Am. Dent. Assoc., 76:772, 1968.

Renstrup, G., et al.: Ten year study of oral leukoplakia. Tandlaegebladet, 72:430, 1968.

LICHEN PLANUS – PEMPHIGUS (See pages 70 and 71.)

Shklar, G., and McCarthy, P. L.: The oral lesions of lichen planus. Oral Surg., *14*:164, 1961.

Whitten, J. B., Jr.: Intraoral lichen planus simplex: An ultrastructure study. J. Periodontol., *41*:261, 1970.

Andreasen, J. O.: Oral lichen planus. I. A clinical evaluation of 115 cases. Oral Surg., 25:31, 1968.

Cooke, B. E. D.: Diagnosing features of pemphigus affecting the oral mucosa. J. Dent. Res., 40:1281, 1961.

Lever, W. F.: Pemphigus. Medicine, 32:1, 1953.

HERPES – MONILIASIS – APHTHOUS ULCERS (See pages 72 and 73.)

Scott, T. F. M., Steigman, A. J., and Convey, J. H.: Acute infectious gingivostomatitis: Etiology, epidemiology, and clinical picture of a common disorder caused by virus of herpes simplex. J.A.M.A., *117*:999, 1941.

Ship, I. I., Brightman, V. J., and Laster, L. L.: The patient with recurrent aphthous ulcers and the patient with recurrent herpes labialis. A study of two population samples. J. Am. Dent. Assoc., 75:645, 1967.

Scott, T. M.: Herpetic stomatitis. J. Dent. Res., 29:647, 1950.

Lehner, T.: Oral thrush, or acute pseudomembranous candidiasis. A clinicopathologic study of forty-four cases. Oral Med., *18*:27, 1964.

Cohen, L.: Oral candidiasis. Oral Surg., 20:316, 1965.

Lehner, T.: Chronic candidiasis. Br. Dent. J., *116*:539, 1964.

Francis, T. C.: Recurrent aphthous stomatitis and Behçet's disease. Oral Surg., 30:476, 1970.

VITAMIN DEFICIENCY (See page 74.)

Mann, A. W., Spies, T. D., and Springer, M.: The oral manifestations of vitamin B complex deficiencies. J. Dent. Res., 20:269, 1941.

Crandon, J. H., Lund, C. C., and Dill, D. B.: Experimental human scurvy. New Engl. J. Med., 223:353, 1940.

Hodges, R. E., et al.: Experimental scurvy in man. Am. J. Clin. Nutr., 22:535, 1969.

Medina, C. A.: Oral manifestations of vitamin deficiencies. Oral Surg., 9:1060, 1956.

Waerhaug, J.: Effect of C-avitaminosis on the supporting structures of the teeth. J. Periodontol., 29:87, 1958.

Glickman, I., and Dines, M.: Effect of increased ascorbic acid blood levels on the ascorbic acid level in treated and nontreated gingiva. J. Dent. Res., 42:1152, 1963.

ALLERGY – ABRASION – BURN (See page 75.)

Martin, J., Bishop, J., Guentherman, R., and Dorman, H.: Cellular response of gingiva to prolonged application of dilute hydrogen peroxide. J. Periodontol., 39:208, 1968.

Koch, G., and Lindhe, J.: The effect of supervised oral hygiene on the gingiva of children. J. Periodont. Res., 2:64, 1967.

RADIOGRAPHIC APPEARANCE — PERIODONTITIS (See pages 76–83.)

Bender, I. B., and Seltzer, S.: Roentgenographic and direct observation of experimental lesions in bone. I. J. Am. Dent. Assoc., 62:152, 1961.

Bender, I. B., and Seltzer, S.: Roentgenographic and direct observation of experimental lesions in bone. II. J. Am. Dent. Assoc., 62:708, 1961.

Parfitt, G. J.: An investigation of the normal variations in alveolar bone trabeculations. Oral Surg., 15:1453, 1962.

Patur, B., and Glickman, I.: Roentgenographic evaluation of alveolar bone changes in periodontal disease. Dent. Clin. North Am., March, 1960, p. 47.

Prichard, J. F.: The role of the roentgenogram in the diagnosis and prognosis of periodontal disease. Oral Surg., 14:182, 1961.

Ramadan, A. B. E., and Mitchell, D. F.: A roentgenographic study of experimental bone destruction. Oral Surg., 15:934, 1962.

Regan, J. E., and Mitchell, D. F.: Roentgenographic and dissection measurements of alveolar crest height. J. Am. Dent. Assoc., 66:356, 1963.

Van der Linden, L. W. J., and Van Aken, J.: The periodontal ligament in the roentgenogram. J. Periodontol., 41:243, 1970.

PERIODONTOSIS (See pages 84–87.)

Glickman, I.: Periodontosis: A critical evaluation. J. Am. Dent. Assoc., 44:706, 1952.

Gottlieb, B.: Etiology and therapy of alveolar pyorrhea. Zschr. f. Stomatol., 18:59, 1920.

Gottlieb, B.: The new concept of periodontoclasia. J. Periodontol., 17:7, 1946.

Kaslick, R. S., and Chasens, A. I.: Periodontosis with periodontitis: A study involving young adult males. Part I. Review of the literature and incidence in a military population. Oral Surg., 25:305, 1968.

Orban, B., and Weinmann, J. P.: Diffuse atrophy of the alveolar bone (periodontosis). J. Periodontol., 13:31, 1942.

Shroff, F. R.: The behavior of collagen fibers in some types of periodontal disease. Oral Surg., 6:1202, 1953.

PATHOLOGIC MIGRATION — DRIFTING — TOOTH MOBILITY (See pages 88–91.)

Hirschfeld, I.: The dynamic relationship between pathologically migrating teeth and inflammatory tissue in periodontal pockets: A clinical study. J. Periodontol., 4:35, 1933.

Mühlemann, H. R.: Tooth mobility: A review of clinical aspects and research findings. J. Periodontol., 38:686, 1967.

O'Leary, T. J.: Tooth mobility. Dent. Clin. North Am., 13:567, 1969.

ALVEOLAR MUCOSA — HARD PALATE (See pages 92 and 93.)

Meyer, J., and Gerson, S. J.: A comparison of human palatal and buccal mucosa. Periodontics, 2:284, 1964.

Orban, B., and Sicher, H.: The oral mucosa. J. Dent. Educ., 10:94, 1945.

VESTIBULE (See pages 94 and 95.)

Hileman, A. C.: Surgical repositioning of vestibule and frenums in periodontal disease. J. Am. Dent. Assoc., 55:676, 1957.

Hilming, F., and Jervoe, P.: Surgical extension of vestibular depth. On the results in various regions of the mouth in periodontal patients. Tandlaegebladet, 74:329, 1970.

RETROMOLAR AREA — MANDIBLE (See pages 96 and 97.)

Clarke, M. A., and Bueltmann, K. W.: Anatomical considerations in periodontal surgery. J. Periodontol., 42:610, 1971.

Craddock, F. W.: Retromolar region of the mandible. J. Am. Dent. Assoc., 47:453, 1953.

Haines, R. W., and Barrett, S. G.: The structure of the mouth in the mandibular molar region. J. Prosthet. Dent., 9:962, 1969.

CEMENTUM — CEMENTICLES (See pages 100 and 101.)

Masters, D. H., and Hoskins, S. W.: Projection of cervical enamel into molar furcations. J. Periodontol., 35:49, 1964.

Mikola, O. J., and Bauer, W. H.: "Cementicles" and fragments of cementum in the periodontal membrane. Oral Surg., 2:1063, 1949.

Gottlieb, B.: Continuous deposition of cementum. J. Am. Dent. Assoc., 30:842, 1943.

Henry, J. L., and Weinmann, J. P.: The pattern of resorption and repair of human cementum. J. Am. Dent. Assoc., 42:270, 1951.

Gottlieb, B., and Orban, B.: Biology and pathology of the tooth and its supporting mechanism. Trans. and Ed. by M. Diamond, New York, The Macmillan Co., 1938, p. 70.

ROOT EXPOSURE — CARIES (See pages 102 and 103.)

Bass, C. C.: A previously undescribed demonstrable pathologic condition in exposed cementum and the underlying dentine. Oral Surg., 4:641, 1951.

Herting, H. C.: Electron microscope studies of the cementum surface structures of periodontally healthy and diseased teeth. J. Dent. Res., *46*:1247, 1967.

Selvig, K. A.: Biological changes at the tooth-saliva interface in periodontal disease. J. Dent. Res., *48*:846, 1969.

PERIODONTAL LIGAMENT FIBERS (See pages 104 and 105.)

Fullmer, H. M.: A histochemical study of periodontal disease in the maxillary alveolar processes of 135 autopsies. J. Periodontol., *32*:206, 1961.

Bien, S. M.: Hydrodynamic damping of tooth movement. J. Dent. Res., *45*:907, 1966.

Ciancio, S. C., Neiders, M. E., and Hazen, S. P.: The principal fibers of the periodontal ligament. Periodontics, *5*:76, 1967.

Coolidge, E. D.: The thickness of the human periodontal membrane. J. Am. Dent. Assoc., *24*:1260, 1937.

Fullmer, H. M.: A critique of normal connective tissues of the periodontium and some alterations with periodontal disease. J. Dent. Res., *41*:223, 1962.

Parfitt, G. J.: The Physical Analysis of Tooth Supporting Structures. *In*: The Mechanisms of Tooth Support. Bristol, J. Wright and Sons, Ltd., 1967, p. 154.

PERIODONTITIS – FIBROTIC GINGIVA (See pages 106 and 107.)

Hock, J., and Niki, K.: A vital microscopy study of the morphology of normal and inflamed gingiva. J. Periodont. Res., *6*:81, 1971.

Melcher, A. H.: The pathogenesis of chronic gingivitis. II. The effect of inflammatory changes in the corium of the overlying epithelium. Dent. Pract., Dent. Rec., *13*:50, 1962.

PERIODONTAL POCKETS (See pages 108 and 109.)

Nuckolls, J., and Dienstein, B., in collab. with Bell, D. G., and Rule, R. W., Jr.: The periodontal lesion. The development of the lesion and the establishment and treatment of the periodontal pocket. J. Periodontol., *21*:7, 1950.

Thilander, H.: Some structural changes in periodontal disease. Dent. Pract., Dent. Rec., *11*:191, 1961.

PERIODONTITIS – SIMPLE AND COMPOUND (See pages 110 and 111.)

Box, H. K.: Twelve Periodontal Studies. Toronto, Canada, The University of Toronto Press, 1940.

Theilade, J.: An evaluation of the reliability of radiographs in the measurement of bone loss in periodontal disease. J. Periodontol., *31*:143, 1960.

PATHWAY OF INFLAMMATION (See pages 112–119.)

Weinmann, J. P.: Progress of gingival inflammation into the supporting structures of the teeth. J. Periodontol., *12*:71, 1941.

Macapanpan, L. C., and Weinmann, J. P.: The influence of injury to the periodontal membrane on the spread of gingival inflammation. J. Dent. Res., *33*:263, 1954.

Glickman, I., and Smulow, J. B.: Effect of excessive occlusal forces upon the pathway of gingival inflammation in humans. J. Periodontol., *36*:141, 1965.

PERIODONTITIS – BUCCO-LINGUAL VIEW (See pages 120 and 121.)

Akiyoshi, M., and Mori, K.: Marginal periodontitis: A histological study of the incipient stage. J. Periodontol., *38*:45, 1967.

Melcher, A. H.: The pathogenesis of chronic gingivitis. I. The spread of the inflammatory process. Dent. Pract., Dent. Rec., *13*:2, 1962.

PERIODONTITIS – MESIO-DISTAL VIEW (See pages 122 and 123.)

Massler, M., Mühlemann, H. R., and Schour, I.: Relation of gingival inflammation to alveolar crest resorption. J. Dent. Res., *32*:704, 1963.

MESIAL MIGRATION (See pages 128 and 129.)

Black, G. V.: Work on Operative Dentistry with which His Special Dental Pathology is Combined. 4 vols., Vol. 1. Pathology of the Hard Tissues of Teeth; Oral Diagnosis. 8th Edition, Chicago, Medico-Dental Publishing Co., 1948, p. 389.

Stein, G., and Weinmann, J. P.: The physiologic movement of the teeth. Ztschr. f. Stomatol., *23*:733, 1925.

Biggerstaff, R. H.: The anterior migration of dentitions and anterior crowding: A review. Angle Orthodont., *37*:227, 1967.

DISTRIBUTION OF FORCES (See pages 130 and 131.)

Picton, D. C. A.: On the part played by the socket in tooth support. Arch. Oral Biol., *10*:945, 1965.

BUTTRESSING BONE (See pages 132 and 133.)

Parfitt, G. J.: An investigation of the normal variations in alveolar bone trabeculation. Oral Surg., *15*:1453, 1962.

Glickman, I., and Smulow, J. B.: Buttressing bone formation in the periodontium. J. Periodontol., *36*:365, 1965.

INFRABONY POCKETS (See pages 134 and 135.)

Carranza, F. A., Jr., and Glickman, I.: Some observations of the microscopic features of infrabony pockets. J. Periodontol., *28*:33, 1957.

Glickman, I., and Smulow, J. B.: Effect of excessive occlusal forces upon the pathway of gingival inflammation in humans. J. Periodontol., 36:141, 1965.

World Workshop in Periodontics, Edited by Ramfjord, S. P., Kerr, A., and Ash, M. Ann Arbor, Michigan, University of Michigan, 1966, p. 272.

Prichard, J.: The infrabony technique as a predictable procedure. J. Periodontol., 28:202, 1957.

TRAUMA FROM OCCLUSION – RADIOGRAPHIC APPEARANCE (See pages 136 and 137.)

Carranza, F. A., and Erausquin, R.: First periodontal findings. Rev. Odont., 27:485, 1939. Buenos Aires, Argentina.

TRAUMA FROM OCCLUSION (See pages 138–145.)

Glickman, I., and Smulow, J. B.: Adaptive alterations in the periodontium of the rhesus monkey in chronic trauma from occlusion. J. Periodontol., 39:101, 1968.

Glickman, I., and Smulow, J. B.: Further observations on the effects of trauma from occlusion in humans. J. Periodontol., 38:280, 1967.

Glickman, I., Stein, R. S., and Smulow, J. B.: The effect of increased functional forces upon the periodontium of splinted and non-splinted teeth. J. Periodontol., 32:290, 1961.

Larato, D. C.: Intrabony defects in the dry human skull. J. Periodontol., 41:496, 1970.

Prichard, J. F.: Periodontal Surgery. Practical Dental Monographs. Chicago, Year Book Publishers, Inc., Nov., 1961, pp. 16–19.

Wentz, F. M., Jarabak, J., and Orban, B.: Experimental occlusal trauma imitating cuspal interferences. J. Periodontol., 29:117, 1958.

ZONES OF IRRITATION AND CO-DESTRUCTION (See pages 146 and 147.)

Glickman, I., and Smulow, J. B.: The combined effects of inflammation and trauma from occlusion in periodontitis. Int. Dent. J., 19:393, 1969.

FURCATION INVOLVEMENT (See pages 148–151.)

Easley, J. R., and Drennan, G. A.: Morphological classification of the furca. J. Can. Dent. Assoc., 35:104, 1969.

Glickman, I.: Bifurcation involvement in periodontal disease. J. Am. Dent. Assoc., 40:528, 1950.

Larato, D. C.: Furcation involvements: Incidence and distribution. J. Periodontol., 41:499, 1970.

Parfitt, G. J.: An investigation of the normal variations in alveolar bone trabeculation. Oral Surg., 15:1453, 1962.

Van der Linden, L. W. J., and Van Aken, J.: The periodontal ligament in the roentgenogram. J. Periodontol., 41:243, 1970.

PERIODONTAL-PULPAL INTERRELATIONSHIPS (See pages 152–155.)

Rubach, W. C., and Mitchell, D. F.: Periodontal disease, accessory canals and pulp pathosis. J. Periodontol., 36:34, 1965.

Mazur, B., and Massler, M.: Influence of periodontal disease on the dental pulp. Oral Surg., 17:592, 1964.

Ross, I. F.: The relation between periodontal and pulpal disorders. J. Am. Dent. Assoc., 84:134, 1972.

Stallard, R. E.: Periodontal disease and its relationship to pulpal pathology. Parodont. Acad. Rev., 2:80, 1968.

Seltzer, S., Bender, I. B., and Ziontz, M.: The interrelationship of pulp and periodontal disease. Oral Surg., 16:1474, 1963.

Simring, M., and Goldberg, M.: The pulpal pocket approach: Retrograde periodontitis. J. Periodontol., 35:22, 1964.

EXPERIMENTAL PATHOLOGY

AGE CHANGES IN THE PERIODONTIUM (See pages 160–162.)

Gilmore, N. D., and Glickman, I.: Some age changes in the periodontium of the albino mouse. J. Dent. Res., 38:1195, 1959.

Cohn, S. A.: Development of the molar teeth in the albino mouse. Am. J. Anat., 101:295, 1957.

Baer, P. N., and Bernick, S.: Age changes in the periodontium of the mouse. Oral Surg., 10:430, 1958.

SYSTEMIC ALTERATION OF ALVEOLAR BONE (See pages 162 and 163.)

Glickman, I.: Effects of acute starvation upon the apposition of alveolar bone associated with the extraction of functional antagonists. J. Dent. Res., 24:155, 1945.

Glickman, I., and Wood, H.: Bone histology in periodontal disease. J. Dent. Res., 21:35, 1942.

Irving, J. T.: Factors concerning bone loss associated with periodontal disease. J. Dent. Res., 49:262, 1970.

VITAMIN C DEFICIENCY (See pages 164–167.)

Glickman, I.: Acute vitamin C deficiency and periodontal disease. I. The periodontal tissues of the guinea pig in acute vitamin C deficiency. J. Dent. Res., 27:9, 1948.

Glickman, I.: Acute vitamin C deficiency and the periodontal tissues. II. The effect of acute vitamin C deficiency upon the response of the periodontal tissues of the guinea pig to artificially induced inflammation. J. Dent. Res., 27:201, 1948.

Turesky, S., and Glickman, I.: Histochemical evaluation of gingival healing in experimental animals on adequate and vitamin C deficient diets. J. Dent. Res., 33:273, 1954.

Boyle, P. E., Bessey, O. A., and Wolbach, S. B.: Experimental production of the diffuse alveolar bone atrophy type of periodontal disease by diets deficient in ascorbic acid. J. Am. Dent. Assoc., 24:1768, 1937.

DIABETES (See pages 168 and 169.)

Glickman, I.: The periodontal structures in experimental diabetes. N. Y. J. Dent., 16:226, 1946.

Shklar, G., Cohen, M. M., and Yerganian, G.: A histopathologic study of periodontal disease in the Chinese hamster with hereditary diabetes. J. Periodontol., 33:14, 1962.

DIABETES AND OCCLUSAL FORCES (See pages 170 and 171.)

Glickman, I., Smulow, J. B., and Moreau, J.: Effect of alloxan diabetes upon the periodontal response to excessive occlusal forces. J. Periodontol., 37:146, 1966.

Cohen, B., and Fosdick, L. S.: Chemical studies in periodontal disease. VI. The glycogen content of gingival tissue in alloxan diabetes. J. Dent. Res., 29:48, 1950.

DIABETES AND PERIODONTAL HEALING (See pages 172 and 173.)

Glickman, I., Smulow, J. B., and Moreau, J.: Postsurgical periodontal healing in alloxan diabetes. J. Periodontol., 38:93, 1967.

Cahill, G. F., Jr., Vance, V. K., and Urrutia, G.: In vitro metabolism of glucose by adrenals from normal and alloxan diabetic rats. Diabetes, 11:318, 1962.

COLD-STRESSED PERIODONTAL TISSUES (See pages 174 and 175.)

Shklar, G., and Glickman, I.: The effect of cold as a stressor agent upon the periodontium of albino rats. Oral Surg., 12:1311, 1959.

Sellers, E. A.: Adaptation and related phenomena in rats exposed to cold. Rev. Canad. Biol., 16:175, 1957.

Selye, H.: The general adaptation syndrome and diseases of adaptation. J. Allergy, 17:231, 1946.

Shklar, G., and Glickman, I.: The periodontium and salivary glands in the alarm reaction. J. Dent. Res., 32:773, 1953.

CORTISONE (See pages 176 and 177.)

Glickman, I., Stone, I., and Chawla, T. N.: The effect of the systemic administration of cortisone upon the periodontium of white mice. J. Periodontol., 24:161, 1953.

Shklar, G.: The effect of adrenalectomy and cortisone replacement on the periodontium of the rat. Periodontics, 3:239, 1965.

CORTISONE MODIFIED BY ESTROGEN (See pages 178 and 179.)

Glickman, I., and Shklar, G.: Modification of the effect of cortisone upon alveolar bone by the systemic administration of estrogen. J. Periodontol., 25:231, 1954.

Nutlay, A. G., Bhaskar, S. N., Weinmann, J. P., and Budy, A. M.: The effect of estrogen on the gingiva and alveolar bone of molars in rats and mice. J. Dent. Res., 33:115, 1954.

ESTROGEN (See pages 180 and 181.)

Glickman, I., and Shklar, G.: The steroid hormones and tissues of the periodontium. Oral Surg., 8:1179, 1955.

Shklar, G., and Glickman, I.: The effect of estrogenic hormone on the periodontium of white mice. J. Periodontol., 27:16, 1956.

OVARIECTOMY (See pages 182 and 183.)

Piroshaw, N., and Glickman, I.: The effect of ovariectomy upon the tissues of the periodontium and skeletal bones. Oral Surg., 10:133, 1957.

Glickman, I., and Quintarelli, J.: Further observations regarding the effects of ovariectomy upon the tissues of the periodontium. J. Periodontol., 31:31, 1960.

OSTEOLATHYRISM (See pages 184 and 185.)

Glickman, I., Selye, H., and Smulow, J. B.: Systemic factors that influence the manifestations of osteolathyrism in the periodontium. J. Dent. Res., 42:835, 1963.

Selye, H.: Lathyrism. Rev. Canad. Biol., 16:3, 1957.

Gardner, A. F.: Influence of injury and adaptation of the periodontal ligament to pathologic changes during experimental lathyrism. J. Periodontol., 30:253, 1959.

Krikos, G. A.: The role of mechanical stress in experimental lathyrism. J. Dent. Res., 40:645, 1961.

CALCIPHYLAXIS (See pages 186 and 187.)

Glickman, I., Selye, H., and Smulow, J. B.: Reduction by calciphylaxis of the effects of chronic dihydrotachysterol overdose upon the periodontium. J. Dent. Res., 44:734, 1965.

Selye, H.: Calciphylaxis. Chicago, University of Chicago Press, 1962.

Moskow, B. S., and Baden, E.: The effect of chronic dihydrotachysterol overdosage on the tissues of the periodontium. A preliminary report. Periodontics, 2:277, 1964.

DILANTIN HYPERPLASIA (See pages 188 and 189.)

Ishikawa, J., and Glickman, I.: Gingival response to the systemic administration of sodium diphenyl hydantoin (Dilantin) in cats. J. Periodontol., 32:149, 1961.

King, J. D.: Experimental production of gingival hyperplasia in ferrets given "Epanutin'" (sodium diphenylhydantoinate). Brit. J. Exper. Path., 33:491, 1952.

Van der Kwast, A. M.: Speculations regarding the nature of gingival hyperplasia due to diphenylhydantoin sodium. Acta Med. Scandinav., *153*:399, 1956.

BUTTRESSING BONE FORMATION (See pages 190 and 191.)

Glickman, I., and Smulow, J. B.: Buttressing bone formation in the periodontium. J. Periodontol., *36*:365, 1965.
Wentz, F. M., Jarabak, J., and Orban, B.: Experimental occlusal trauma imitating cuspal interferences. J. Periodontol., *29*:117, 1958.

SPLINTS AND OCCLUSAL FORCES (See pages 192 and 193.)

Glickman, I., Stein, R. S., and Smulow, J. B.: The effect of increased functional forces upon the periodontium of splinted and non-splinted teeth. J. Periodontol., *32*:290, 1961.
Weinberg, L. A.: Force distribution in splinted anterior teeth. Oral Surg., *10*:484, 1957.
Bhaskar, S. N., and Orban, B.: Experimental occlusal trauma. J. Periodontol., *26*:270, 1955.
Glickman, I., and Weiss, L.: Role of trauma from occlusion in initiation of periodontal pocket formation in experimental animals. J. Periodontol., *26*:14, 1955.
Ewen, S. J., and Stahl, S. S.: The response of the periodontium to chronic gingival irritation and long-term tilting forces in adult dogs. Oral Surg., *15*:1426, 1962.

PATHWAY OF INFLAMMATION (See pages 194 and 195.)

Glickman, I., and Smulow, J. B.: Alterations in the pathway of gingival inflammation into the underlying tissues induced by excessive occlusal forces. J. Periodontol., *33*:7, 1962.
Glickman, I.: Occlusion and the periodontium. J. Dent. Res., *46*:53, 1967.

CHRONIC TRAUMA FROM OCCLUSION (See pages 196 and 197.)

Waerhaug, J., and Hansen, E. R.: Periodontal changes incident to prolonged occlusal overload in monkeys. Acta Odontol. Scand., *24*:91, 1966.
Glickman, I., and Smulow, J. B.: Adaptive alterations in the periodontium of the rhesus monkey in chronic trauma from occlusion. J. Periodontol., *39*:101, 1968.
Wentz, F. M., Jarabak, J., and Orban, B.: Experimental occlusal trauma imitating cuspal interferences. J. Periodontol., *29*:117, 1958.

HEALING AFTER MUCOGINGIVAL SURGERY (See pages 198 and 199.)

Glickman, I., Smulow, J. B., O'Brien, T., and Tannen, R.: Healing of the periodontium following mucogingival surgery. Oral Surg., *16*:530, 1963.
Ramfjord, S. P., and Costich, E. R.: Healing after exposure of periosteum on the alveolar process. J. Periodontol., *39*:199, 1968.
Waerhaug, J.: Review of Cohen: "Role of Periodontal Surgery." J. Dent. Res., *50*:219, 1971.
Wilderman, M. N.: Exposure of bone in periodontal surgery. Dent. Clin. North Am., March, 1964, p. 23.

MUCOGINGIVAL SURGERY AND OCCLUSAL FORCES (See pages 200 and 201.)

Glickman, I., Smulow, J. B., Vogel, G., and Passamonti, G.: The effect of occlusal forces on healing following mucogingival surgery. J. Periodontol., *37*:319, 1966.
Wilderman, M., Wentz, F. M., and Orban, B. J.: Histogenesis of repair after mucogingival surgery. J. Periodontol., *31*:283, 1960.
Arnold, N. R., and Hatchett, C. M., Jr.: A comparative investigation of two mucogingival surgical methods. J. Periodontol., *33*:129, 1962.
Carranza, F. A., Jr., and Carraro, J. J.: Mucogingival techniques in periodontal surgery. J. Periodontol., *41*:294, 1970.

BONE GRINDING AND HEALING (See page 202.)

Lobene, R., and Glickman, I.: The response of alveolar bone to grinding with rotary diamond stones. J. Periodontol., *34*:105, 1963.
Kohler, C. A., and Ramfjord, S. P.: Healing of gingival mucoperiosteal flaps. Oral Surg., *13*:89, 1960.

ELECTROSURGERY AND HEALING (See page 203.)

Glickman, I., and Imber, L. R.: Comparison of gingival resection with electrosurgery and periodontal knives—A biometric and histologic study. J. Periodontol., *41*:142, 1970.
Pope, J. W., Gargiulo, A. W., Staffileno, H., and Levy, S.: Effects of electrosurgery on wound healing in dogs. Periodontics, *6*:30, 1968.
Malone, W. F., and Manning, J. L.: Electrosurgery in restorative dentistry. J. Prosthet. Dent., *20*:417, 1968.

Index